The First-Time Mom's Guide to Pregnancy

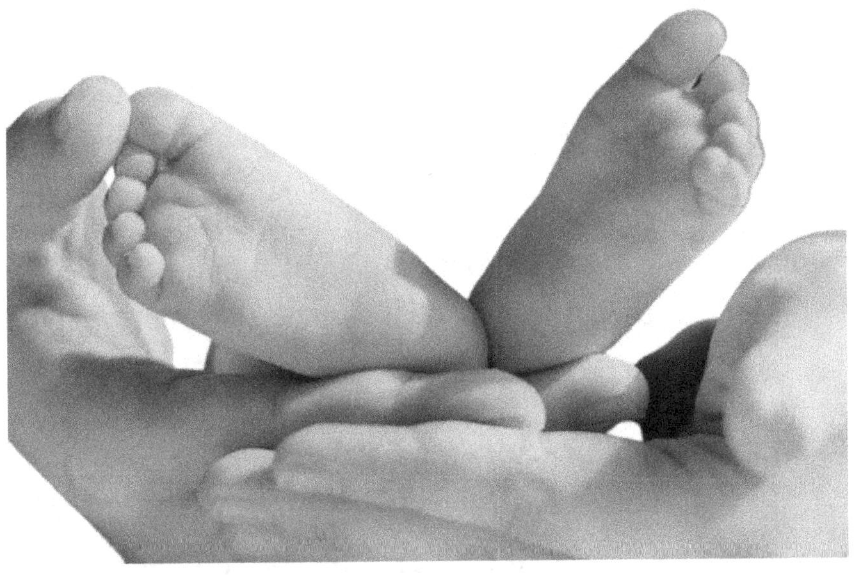

Glowing Through Pregnancy

Laura Walker

Table of Content

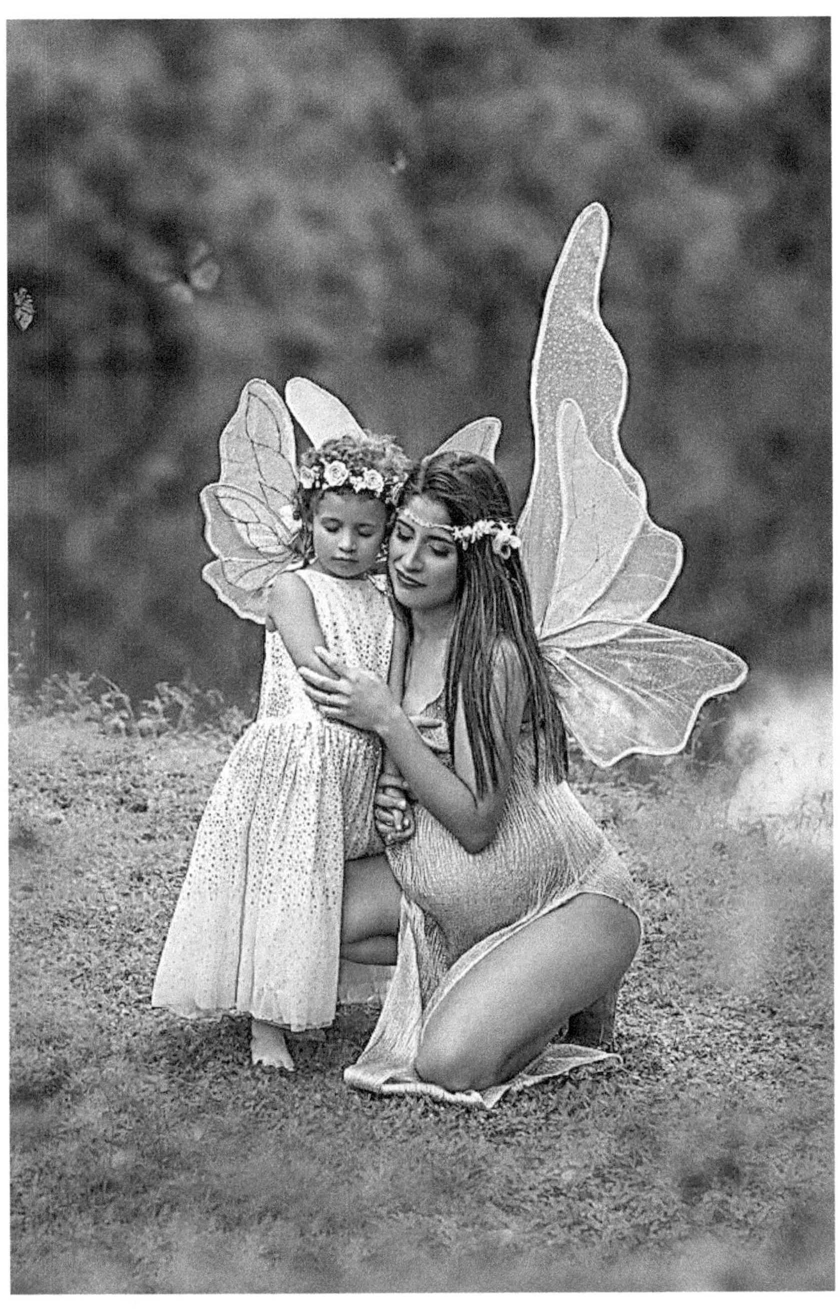

Introduction

In the realm of life's greatest miracles, few experiences compare to the transformative journey of motherhood. From the first flutter of life within to the awe-inspiring moments of childbirth, it is a remarkable adventure that has captivated generations of women. It is a tale of strength, vulnerability, love, and growth, woven together with countless unique stories that echo across time.

Imagine a young woman, her heart overflowing with anticipation, as she embarks on this sacred path. Let us follow her footsteps, her hopes, her fears, and her triumphs, as we delve into the journey and experiences of an expectant mother. Her story reflects the universal tapestry of motherhood, resonating with every woman who has ever embraced this extraordinary chapter in her life.

As an expectant mother you stand at the precipice of change, your body and soul is alive with the knowledge of a tiny, wondrous life growing within you. The discovery of your pregnancy unfolds like a delicate secret, shared first with her partner, and later with loved ones. Emotions intermingle—a symphony of joy, disbelief, and nervous anticipation—creating a deep bond between mother and child, even before your eyes meet.

As the days turn into weeks, your body begins to transform, gently nudging you to accept the extraordinary nature of this voyage. The first trimester brings its own unique set of challenges, as you navigate the unpredictable terrain of morning sickness, fatigue, and hormonal fluctuations. Yet, amidst the discomfort, you discover a newfound resilience and a fierce protectiveness that fuels your determination to provide the best possible environment for your growing child. In the second trimester, you find yourself marveling at the miracle unfolding before your eyes. With each passing day, the baby's movements grow stronger, transforming from delicate flutters to playful kicks. You delight in the secret communication between you and your baby, cherishing this special bond that transcends words.

Simultaneously, you immerse yourself in the world of prenatal care, seeking expert guidance to ensure your baby's well-being. From choosing a trusted healthcare provider to understanding the importance of a balanced diet and exercise, you embrace your role as the guardian of this precious life. Prenatal classes become a rite of passage, connecting you with other expectant mothers, each with their own stories of hope, dreams, and the occasional midnight craving.

With the third trimester comes a flurry of activity, as you lovingly prepare your home for the arrival of your little one. The nesting instinct takes hold, driving you to create a sanctuary of warmth, comfort, and security. From selecting the perfect crib to meticulously arranging tiny garments, you pour your heart into every detail, eagerly anticipating the day you will hold your baby in your arms.

Alongside the practical preparations, you immerse yourself in the wealth of knowledge available. You read books on childbirth, attends birthing classes, and explores various birthing options, seeking to empower yourself with the knowledge necessary to make informed decisions. You realize that, ultimately, your experience of childbirth will be as unique as your journey itself. As the final days of pregnancy draw near, you experience a symphony of emotions—excitement, apprehension, and a profound sense of wonder. The momentous day arrives, and you are enveloped in a whirlwind of emotions as your body works in harmony with nature, bringing forth new life.

As the final moments approach, a crescendo of emotions fills the room. With one final push, you bring forth your greatest creation—a tiny, fragile being—your child. The room erupts with a chorus of tears, laughter, and the first cries of a newborn. In that instant, your heart expands to accommodate a love so profound, it defies description.

With the birth of your child, you begin a dance that will last a lifetime—the intricate steps of motherhood. You embrace sleepless nights and endless diaper changes with grace and tenderness. You discover the incredible power of your nurturing touch, soothing your baby's cries and fostering an unbreakable bond.

Each day brings new lessons and challenges as you navigate the complexities of breastfeeding, comforting a fussy baby, and adapting to the rhythm of your child's needs. You rely on your intuition, honed by the connection forged during pregnancy, and draws strength from the community of mothers who share your journey. As the days turn into weeks, and weeks into months, you witness the miraculous growth and development of your child. You marvel at each milestone—the first smile, the first word, the first steps—as your heart swells with pride and joy. In the face of fatigue and self-doubt, you find solace in the knowledge that you are part of an unbroken lineage of mothers who have nurtured, guided, and loved their children since time immemorial.

As your child grows, you discover that motherhood is an ever-evolving journey. You learn to adapt to the changing needs of your child, finding balance between nurturing and guiding, protecting and letting go. Alongside the challenges, you experience the immeasurable rewards of witnessing your child flourish into a unique individual, guided by the love and guidance you offer.

In the tapestry of motherhood, an expectant mother story is but one thread woven into a grand design. She joins the ranks of countless women who have embarked on this sacred journey, each with their own experiences, triumphs, and challenges. Together, they form a collective strength, a sisterhood of mothers who support and uplift one another.

The journey and experiences of an expectant mother encompass the essence of life itself—its beauty, fragility, and boundless capacity for love. From the seed of life to the miracle of birth and beyond, the expectant mother's story echoes throughout time, resonating with every woman who has embarked on this extraordinary voyage.

Through the challenges, sacrifices, and moments of sheer wonder, she discovers the depths of her own strength and the limitless power of her love. And as she embraces the role of motherhood, she becomes a guardian of life's most precious gift—a child who will forever carry the imprints of her love and the legacy of her journey.

In the pages of this book, we embark on this timeless odyssey together, celebrating the diverse stories, triumphs, and lessons of expectant mothers from all walks of life. May their experiences inspire, empower, and illuminate the path for every woman who embarks on the extraordinary adventure of motherhood.

Chapter 1

The Miracle of Motherhood: A Journey of Love and Wonder

Motherhood—a word that carries within it the essence of love, sacrifice, and boundless joy. It is a transformative journey, an odyssey of emotions that begins long before your baby takes their first breath. From the moment you discover that tiny life growing within you, a miracle unfolds. Every kick, flutter, and hiccup becomes a testament to the awe-inspiring wonder of creation.

You're sitting in a quiet room, bathed in warm sunlight, as you gently cradle your growing belly. Your heart swells with anticipation and love as you feel the gentle movements of your baby. In those moments, you realize that within you lies a world of possibilities, a tiny being waiting to discover the wonders of life. It is in this realization that the true miracle of motherhood takes hold.

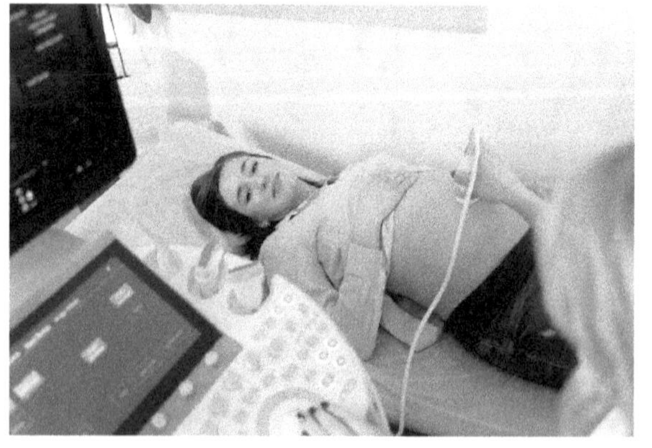

The journey of motherhood begins with the knowledge that you are carrying life within you— a life that is uniquely yours and yet a part of something greater. It is a connection that transcends words, a bond that forms in the quiet depths of your soul. As your baby grows, so does the intensity of this bond. You find yourself daydreaming about their first smile, their first steps, and the countless memories you will create together.

But along with the awe and wonder comes a wave of emotions. From the sheer joy of feeling those first flutters to the vulnerability and uncertainty that accompany the responsibility of nurturing a life, motherhood encompasses a spectrum of feelings. It is perfectly normal to experience moments of overwhelming love, mixed with bouts of anxiety and even doubt. After all, you are about to embark on a journey that will test your limits, challenge your patience, and transform you in ways you never thought possible.

Lying in bed, exhausted after a day filled with swollen feet and backaches. As you close your eyes, you feel a gentle nudge against your ribs. It's your baby, reminding you of their presence and the miracle unfolding within you. In that moment, fatigue dissipates, and you're filled with a sense of purpose and unconditional love. The tiredness fades away as you realize that every discomfort is a small price to pay for the miracle growing inside you.

As your pregnancy progresses, you become attuned to the rhythm of your baby's movements. You realize that they have their own unique personality, even before they take their first breath. Sometimes they dance joyfully, responding to the melodies that fill your days. Other times, they curl up in a quiet cocoon, seeking solace and peace. These moments remind you that you are not alone in this journey. You are a vessel, a protector, and a nurturer—a guardian of this precious life.

The miracle of motherhood extends beyond the physical realm. It is an emotional and spiritual awakening, an opportunity to witness the strength and resilience of the human spirit. It is in the early morning hours when you find yourself sleep-deprived and weary, yet still mustering the energy to comfort your restless baby. It is in the moments when you doubt yourself and question your abilities as a mother, only to find the answer in the smile that lights up your baby's face.

Picture yourself cradling your newborn in your arms, their tiny hand gripping your finger. You gaze into their eyes, and in that fleeting instant, you see a reflection of your love, your hopes, and your dreams. It is a profound connection that transcends time, a bond that signifies the beginning of a lifelong journey together. In those tender moments, you become acutely aware of the depth of your capacity to love and the resilience of your heart.

The miracle of motherhood extends beyond the boundaries of your physical being. It touches every aspect of your life, weaving its way into your relationships, your aspirations, and your sense of self. It is a journey that challenges you to grow, to discover hidden strengths, and to embrace the profound transformation that comes with bringing new life into the world.

In the midst of this miraculous journey, you may encounter moments of vulnerability and self-doubt. The weight of responsibility can feel overwhelming at times, as you navigate the sleepless nights, the endless diaper changes, and the ceaseless demands of caring for a tiny human being. But remember, dear mother, that you are not alone. Reach out to your support network, lean on the wisdom and experience of those who have walked this path before you. They will remind you that you possess an inner resilience and love that knows no bounds.

As you embrace the miracle of motherhood, you also discover the power of selflessness. It is in those quiet acts of sacrifice—the sleep you give up, the dreams you put on hold, the moments of self-care that you forgo—that you realize the depth of your love for your child. Your desires and needs take a backseat as you prioritize the well-being and happiness of this precious soul you hold in your arms.

You may find yourself gazing at your reflection in the mirror, noticing the changes in your body—stretch marks etched across your skin, a softer silhouette that tells the story of your journey. In those moments, allow yourself to feel a sense of awe and reverence for what your body has accomplished. Each mark, each curve is a testament to the miracle of life you have nurtured within. Embrace these physical changes as a badge of honor, a reminder of the incredible strength and resilience that lies within you. But amidst the joys and challenges, it is crucial to remember that you are not only a mother—you are also an individual with dreams, passions, and a unique identity.

The miracle of motherhood does not diminish your essence; rather, it enriches it. As you guide and nurture your child, remember to hold onto the parts of yourself that make you who you are. Pursue your passions, seek moments of self-care, and nurture your own growth. By doing so, you demonstrate to your child the importance of embracing one's authentic self and living a life filled with purpose.

As you embark on this remarkable journey, remember to be kind to yourself. Motherhood is a series of highs and lows, victories and challenges, but you are doing the best you can. Trust your instincts, listen to your heart, and find solace in the knowledge that you are the perfect mother for your child. Each smile, each milestone, each whispered "I love you" will affirm that you are exactly where you are meant to be.

Expectant moms often experience a range of emotions during their pregnancy, from joy and excitement to anxiety and worry. It's important to remember that these feelings are normal and to find ways to embrace the emotional rollercoaster.

How to Manage Emotions as an Expectant Mom

Here are some tips to help expectant moms navigate their emotions during pregnancy:

1. **Acknowledge your feelings:** It's important to recognize and accept your emotions, whether they're positive or negative. Don't feel guilty for feeling anxious or sad; it's a natural part of the process.

2. **Talk to someone:** Share your feelings with your partner, family member, or close friend. Sometimes just talking about what's on your mind can help alleviate some of the anxiety.

3. **Practice self-care:** Take care of yourself physically and mentally. Get enough rest,

eat well, and exercise if your doctor approves. Engage in activities that bring you joy, such as reading, listening to music, or taking a relaxing bath.

4.   **Educate yourself:** Educate yourself about pregnancy and childbirth. This can help alleviate some of the anxiety that comes from the unknown.

5.   **Seek support:** Consider joining a support group for expectant moms. Talking to others who are going through the same thing can be incredibly helpful.

It's normal to feel a range of emotions during pregnancy. By acknowledging your feelings, talking to someone, practicing self-care, educating yourself, and seeking support, you can embrace the emotional rollercoaster and enjoy this special time in your life.

Prenatal bonding activities: Engage in activities that allow you to connect with your baby before birth. Talk to your baby, sing lullabies, or read books aloud. Gentle massages on your belly can also create a soothing connection.

Play soothing music: Play calming and soothing music for your baby. Research suggests that babies can respond to music even before birth. It can be a beautiful way to create a peaceful environment and establish a bond.

Practice mindfulness and meditation: Engage in mindfulness or meditation exercises to create a sense of calm and connection with your baby. Focus on your breathing and visualize positive interactions with your little one.

Bond through touch: Gently stroke your belly and feel your baby's movements. As your pregnancy progresses, you may notice specific patterns of activity. Respond to those movements with gentle touches or softly talking to your baby.

Involve your partner: Encourage your partner to participate in bonding activities as well. They can talk to the baby, read stories, or even accompany you to prenatal appointments. Sharing these experiences can strengthen the bond as a family.

Create a nurturing environment: Prepare the nursery or the space where your baby will be welcomed. Surround yourself with items that hold sentimental value or are associated with positive emotions. This helps create a nurturing atmosphere for both you and your baby.

Attend childbirth education classes: Enroll in childbirth education classes where you can learn about the birthing process and early newborn care. Understanding what to expect can help you feel more connected and confident as you prepare for your baby's arrival.

Establish a routine of self-care: Take care of yourself physically, emotionally, and mentally. Nurturing your own well-being allows you to be in a better position to bond with your baby. Get adequate rest, eat healthily, and engage in activities that bring you joy.

Visualize bonding moments: Take some quiet time each day to visualize positive bonding moments with your baby. Imagine holding them, cuddling, and sharing joyful experiences together. Visualization can help strengthen the emotional connection.

Trust your instincts: Remember that you are already forming a bond with your baby through the experiences and choices you make as an expectant mom. Trust your instincts and embrace the unique connection you have with your little one.

By incorporating these strategies into your routine, you can nurture a strong bond with your baby during pregnancy, setting a foundation for a loving and connected relationship as you move forward into parenthood.

Dear mother, the miracle of motherhood is a tapestry woven with the threads of love, sacrifice, and unwavering devotion. It is a journey that will test your limits, expand your heart, and shape your very essence. Embrace the ups and downs, the tears and laughter, knowing that you are part of something greater—a timeless tradition of love and nurturing that spans generations. As you embark on this sacred path, may you find strength, joy, and a profound sense of purpose in the miracle of motherhood.

Chapter 2

Preparing Your Mind and Body: Nurturing the Sacred Temple Within

As you embark on the journey of motherhood, it becomes essential to prepare not only your physical body but also your mind and spirit. The transformational process of nurturing life within requires a strong foundation—one

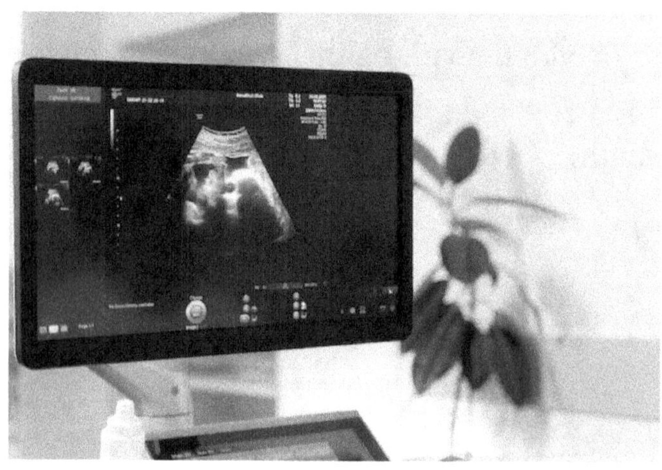

built on self-care, positivity, and a deep connection with your inner self.

In this chapter, we explore the significance of preparing your mind and body, equipping you with the tools to navigate the incredible adventure that lies ahead.

You find yourself sitting in a peaceful garden, the scent of blooming flowers filling the air. The warm rays of the sun envelop you, as you take a deep breath, allowing a sense of calm and serenity to wash over you. In this moment, you recognize the importance of cultivating a positive and nurturing mindset as you prepare to welcome your little one into the world.

Preparing your mind begins with acknowledging the power of thoughts and emotions. Pregnancy, like any transformative journey, can evoke a range of emotions—from excitement and joy to anxiety and fear. It is crucial to create a mental space that fosters positivity and self-belief. Reflect on the beauty of the life growing within you, envision the joys that lie ahead, and embrace the miraculous nature of motherhood.

You may find yourself lying in bed, your mind swirling with worries and doubts. The weight of responsibility may feel overwhelming, as thoughts of the challenges ahead cloud your mind. In those moments, allow yourself to take a deep breath and consciously redirect your thoughts. **Remind yourself of the strength and resilience you possess.** Visualize yourself cradling your baby, surrounded by love and support. By consciously shifting your focus towards positivity, you create a mental landscape that nurtures both you and your growing child.

Nurturing your mind also involves creating space for self-care. As a mother, it is easy to prioritize the needs of others above your own. However, it is essential to remember that your well-being directly impacts your ability to care for your little one. Find moments of solitude and indulge in activities that bring you joy and peace. Whether it's reading a book, taking long walks in nature, practicing yoga, or simply enjoying a warm bath, these moments of self-nurturing replenish your energy and recharge your spirit.

Picture yourself standing in front of a mirror, your body changing with each passing day. It's natural to experience moments of insecurity or frustration as your body adapts to the demands of pregnancy. However, it is crucial to embrace and celebrate the sacred temple that is your body. Each curve, each stretch mark is a testament to the incredible journey you are undertaking. Take a moment to gently caress your growing belly, acknowledging the miracle that lies within. Nurture a sense of gratitude for the vessel that carries life, and let go of societal expectations or self-imposed pressures. By cultivating self-love and acceptance, you create an environment of compassion and reverence within yourself.

The process of preparing your body for the journey of motherhood goes beyond physical fitness—it encompasses nourishment, rest, and overall well-being. Pregnancy nutrition plays a vital role in supporting both your health and the development of your baby. Embrace a balanced and nutritious diet, rich in fruits, vegetables, whole grains, and lean proteins. Listen to your body's cravings and aversions, honoring its unique needs while making mindful choices that promote optimal health for both you and your little one.

You may find yourself in the kitchen, surrounded by colorful ingredients, as you prepare a meal for yourself and your baby. As you chop fresh vegetables and savor the aroma of spices, take a moment to reflect on the nourishment you are providing. Each bite is a gesture of love and care, a testament to the profound connection you share with your unborn child. As you savor each mouthful, imagine the nutrients being absorbed by your body, nourishing your baby's growth and development. Let the act of preparing and consuming food become a sacred ritual, a reminder of the vital role you play in nurturing life.

Rest and relaxation are equally crucial in preparing your body for the miraculous journey of motherhood. Pregnancy places increased demands on your physical and emotional well-being. Honor the importance of restful sleep, allowing your body to rejuvenate and regenerate. Create a soothing bedtime routine, indulge in calming rituals such as reading, gentle stretching, or listening to soothing music.

Prioritize quality sleep, knowing that it is an essential aspect of replenishing your energy reserves and promoting overall health.

Imagine yourself lying on a comfortable bed, surrounded by soft pillows and cozy blankets. As you close your eyes, you feel the weight of the day slowly lifting from your shoulders. In this moment of stillness, allow yourself to fully surrender to the embrace of sleep. Release any lingering worries or anxieties, trusting that the universe is watching over you and your baby. Embrace the restorative power of sleep, knowing that each moment of rest is a gift you give not only to yourself but also to your growing child.

Preparing your mind and body also involves cultivating a deep sense of connection with your inner self and your baby. Take time each day to connect with the life growing within you. Set aside moments of quiet contemplation, placing your hands on your belly, and feeling the gentle movements and kicks. Allow yourself to have intimate conversations with your unborn child, whispering words of love and encouragement. As you forge this bond, you are nurturing not only the physical connection but also a spiritual and emotional connection that will transcend the boundaries of time.

Picture yourself sitting in a serene space, soft music playing in the background. As you close your eyes, you visualize a warm, golden light surrounding your baby and yourself. In this visualization, you send love and positive energy to your little one, creating a profound connection of love and protection. Feel the warmth spreading through your body, enveloping you and your baby in a cocoon of love. By consciously nurturing this spiritual bond, you are laying the foundation for a lifetime of love and connection with your child.

Preparing your mind and body for the journey of motherhood is a sacred and transformative process. By cultivating a positive mindset, practicing self-care, nourishing your body, and fostering a deep connection with your inner self and your baby, you create a strong and resilient foundation. As you embark on this miraculous journey, remember to embrace each moment, trusting in your innate wisdom and capacity to nurture life. You are embarking on a journey of love and self-discovery, and with every step, you are shaping not only your own destiny but also the destiny of the precious life growing within you. Embrace the power of this preparation, knowing that you are creating the best possible environment for yourself and your baby to thrive.

Excitement, Joy and Anticipation for Pregnant Mom

Expectant moms may experience a range of emotions about motherhood, including excitement, joy, and anticipation, as well as anxiety, fear, and uncertainty. Cultivating a positive mindset can help ease anxiety and create a more fulfilling experience. Here are some ways to cultivate a positive mindset towards motherhood:

1. **Focus on the positive:** Make a conscious effort to focus on the positive aspects of motherhood. Surround yourself with supportive people, read positive literature, and visualize joyful experiences with your baby.

2. **Practice self-care:** Taking care of yourself is an important part of developing a positive mindset. Engage in activities that bring you joy, eat healthy, get enough sleep, and exercise if your doctor approves.

3. **Set realistic expectations:** Recognize that motherhood is a journey with both ups and downs. Setting realistic expectations can help you navigate challenges with more ease.

4. **Connect with other expectant or new moms:** Talking with others who are going through the same experience can provide valuable support and perspective.

5. **Educate yourself:** Learning about pregnancy, childbirth, and parenting can help you feel more informed and empowered. Attend childbirth

education classes and seek out reputable sources of information.

6. **Embrace imperfection:** It's normal to make mistakes as a new mom. Embrace imperfection and allow yourself to learn from your experiences.

7. **Practice mindfulness:** Mindfulness techniques, such as deep breathing and meditation, can help you stay present and calm, reducing anxiety and increasing positive feelings.

8. **Talk with your partner:** Having open and honest conversations with your partner about your expectations and feelings can help you both feel more connected and supported.

9. **Trust your instincts:** As a new mom, you will be faced with many decisions. Trusting your instincts and intuition can help you make the best choices for yourself and your baby.

Developing a positive mindset toward motherhood is a process. It takes time, patience, and effort, but the benefits are worth it. By incorporating these strategies into your routine, you can approach motherhood with a sense of calm, confidence, and joy.

Nourishing Your Body and Understanding Pregnancy Nutrition:

Eat a balanced diet: Focus on consuming a variety of nutrient-dense foods, including fruits, vegetables, whole grains, lean proteins, and healthy fats.

Increase your intake of folic acid: Folic acid is a B vitamin that is essential for proper fetal development. It can be found in fortified cereals, leafy green vegetables, and citrus fruits.

1. **Stay hydrated:** Aim to drink at least 8-10 cups of water each day to stay hydrated and support healthy blood flow to the placenta.

2. **Limit your intake of processed foods and added sugars:** These foods can be high in empty calories and may increase your risk of gestational diabetes and other pregnancy complications.

3. **Avoid certain foods:** Avoid raw or undercooked meats, seafood, and eggs, as well as unpasteurized dairy products

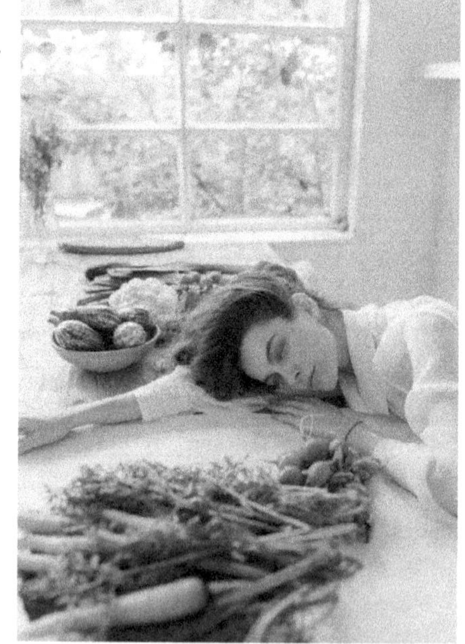

and soft cheeses, as they may increase the risk of foodborne illnesses.

4. **Talk to your healthcare provider about supplements:** In addition to prenatal vitamins, your healthcare provider may recommend other supplements, such as iron or calcium, to support a healthy pregnancy.

5. **Listen to your body:** Pay attention to your hunger and fullness cues, and adjust your food intake as needed. You may find that smaller, more frequent meals throughout the day are more comfortable than larger meals.

6. **Practice mindful eating:** Take time to savor your food and enjoy the experience of eating. This can help you feel more satisfied and prevent overeating.

7. **Keep a food diary:** Keeping a food diary can help you track your nutrient intake and identify areas where you may need to make adjustments.

8. **Attend nutrition education classes:** Attend classes or seek out reputable sources of information to learn more about healthy pregnancy nutrition and how to make informed choices.

By incorporating these strategies into your routine, you can nourish your body and support a healthy pregnancy. Remember, every pregnancy is different, and it's important to work with your healthcare provider to develop a personalized nutrition plan that meets your unique needs.

Exercise and Self-Care during Pregnancy

Embracing exercise and self-care during pregnancy is crucial for maintaining physical and mental well-being. Here's an expert perspective on how to approach exercise and self-care during pregnancy:

Consult with your healthcare provider: Before starting

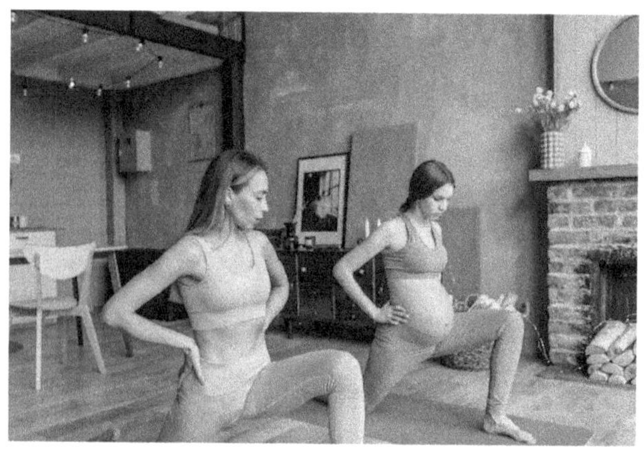

any exercise routine during pregnancy, consult with your healthcare provider or obstetrician. They can provide personalized guidance based on your specific needs and any potential risks or restrictions.

1. **Choose pregnancy-friendly exercises:** Engage in exercises that are safe and suitable for pregnancy. Low-impact activities like walking, swimming,

prenatal yoga, and stationary cycling are generally recommended. These exercises help improve cardiovascular health, strengthen muscles, and promote flexibility.

2. **Listen to your body:** Pay attention to how your body feels during exercise. If something doesn't feel right or causes discomfort, modify or stop the activity. Your body is going through significant changes, so it's important to respect its signals.

3. **Stay hydrated and cool:** Drink plenty of water before, during, and after exercise to stay hydrated. Avoid overheating by exercising in well-ventilated areas, wearing breathable clothing, and taking breaks as needed.

4. **Practice pelvic floor exercises:** Strengthening the pelvic floor muscles can be beneficial during pregnancy and for postpartum recovery. Consult with a healthcare professional or a certified prenatal exercise specialist to learn proper techniques for pelvic floor exercises.

5. **Prioritize self-care:** Pregnancy can be physically and emotionally demanding, so self-care is essential. Make time for activities that help you relax and unwind, such as taking warm baths, getting prenatal massages, practicing mindfulness or meditation, or indulging in hobbies you enjoy.

6.   **Get enough rest:** Pregnancy can cause fatigue, so ensure you're getting enough sleep and rest. Listen to your body and allow yourself to take breaks when needed. Quality sleep is crucial for your overall well-being and the healthy development of your baby.

7.   **Practice stress management techniques:** Pregnancy can come with its share of stress and anxiety. Engage in stress management techniques such as deep breathing exercises, gentle stretching, or engaging in activities that bring you joy and calmness.

8.   **Seek support:** Connect with other expectant moms or join prenatal support groups where you can share experiences, and concerns, and seek advice. Having a support system can help alleviate stress and provide a sense of community.

9.   **Celebrate your body:** Embrace the changes happening in your body and celebrate the incredible journey of pregnancy. Practice positive body image and self-acceptance, recognizing the strength and beauty of your body as it nurtures new life.

Chapter 3
Understanding Prenatal Care and Choosing a Healthcare Provider: Nurturing Your Baby's Journey with Love and Guidance

The moment you discover that you are expecting a baby, an overwhelming surge of emotions rushes through your veins. Excitement, joy, and perhaps a touch of anxiety fill your heart as you embark on the extraordinary journey of motherhood. In this chapter, we delve into the profound significance of prenatal care and the pivotal role of choosing a healthcare provider who will be your guiding light, offering compassion, expertise, and unwavering support. Let us explore this essential aspect of your journey together, as we nurture your baby's growth with love and guidance.

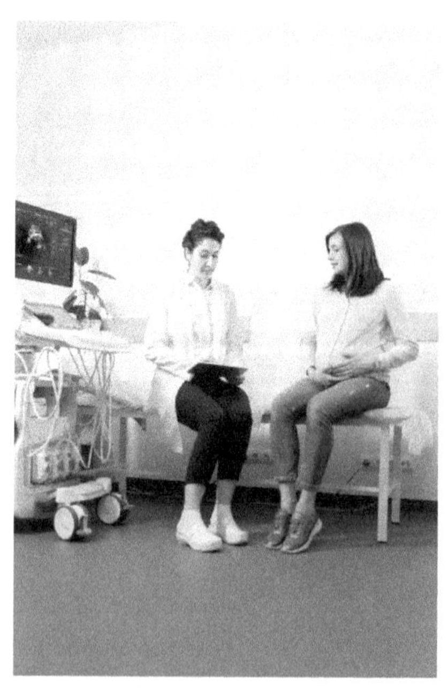

You find yourself in a cozy waiting room, clutching your hands together, your heart fluttering like a delicate butterfly. The room is filled with a mix of anticipation and trepidation, as you await your first prenatal appointment. In this moment, the magnitude of prenatal care becomes clear—the vital lifeline that will safeguard your baby's journey from the very   beginning. Prenatal care is a comprehensive approach to nurturing the well-being of both you and your precious baby. It encompasses a series of medical check-ups, tests, and consultations with healthcare professionals who specialize in the miraculous realm of pregnancy and childbirth. These dedicated individuals will become your guardians, providing essential monitoring, guidance, and reassurance throughout the transformative nine months of gestation.

Choosing a healthcare provider who not only possesses expertise and qualifications but also resonates with your values and honors your unique desires is an indispensable step in your journey. Consider this relatable example: Picture yourself sitting across from a healthcare provider, their eyes filled with warmth and compassion as they attentively listen to your hopes, fears, and dreams for your baby. Their genuine care and willingness to embrace your wishes make you feel seen and cherished. In that precious moment, you know deep within your heart that you have discovered a trusted partner who will walk beside you through every step of this remarkable adventure.

When selecting a healthcare provider, take into account their experience, qualifications, and approach to prenatal care. Seek recommendations from trusted sources, read reviews, and don't hesitate to schedule meetings to assess their compatibility with your needs and preferences. Trust your intuition, for it will guide you towards someone who not only possesses the necessary expertise but also radiates a nurturing and supportive presence.

Once you have chosen your healthcare provider, the journey of prenatal care commences. It encompasses a series of regular check-ups that serve as milestones in your baby's development and provide you with invaluable support and guidance. These appointments become precious moments to connect with the miracle growing within you and receive the nurturing care and expertise of your healthcare provider.

You find yourself in the examination room, your heart pounding with anticipation as you await the first glimpse of your baby. The room is filled with an air of excitement and nervous anticipation. As the gentle sound of the Doppler fills the room, you hold your breath, yearning to hear the enchanting rhythm of your baby's heartbeat. In that miraculous moment, tears of overwhelming joy stream down your face, and a surge of love washes over you. The comforting words and reassuring smile of your healthcare provider remind you that you are not alone on this journey of motherhood.

Prenatal care also entails a series of tests and screenings designed to assess your health and monitor your baby's well-being. These tests may include blood work, ultrasound scans, genetic screenings, and other assessments to ensure that both you and your baby are progressing as expected. While the anticipation and anxiety surrounding these tests may be palpable, remember that they are essential in providing vital information and ensuring the best possible care for you and your precious little one.

You find yourself in a softly lit ultrasound room, the air pregnant with anticipation. You lay on the examination table, your partner by your side, their hand intertwined with yours, a symbol of unwavering support. As the ultrasound technician glides the wand over your belly, a mixture of nervousness and excitement fills the room. And then, like a flickering star in the night sky, your baby appears on the screen—a tiny, perfect being with a beating heart and delicate features. Overwhelmed with awe and emotion, tears of joy spill from your eyes, tracing the path of unconditional love etched in your heart.

In that tender moment, you realize the profound significance of prenatal care. It is not just a series of medical procedures or routine check-ups; it is an act of love, a testament to your devotion as a mother. Prenatal care serves as a protective cocoon, enveloping you and your baby in a web of support and guidance, ensuring that every step of this miraculous journey is nurtured with tenderness.

Choosing a healthcare provider who understands the depth of this emotional tapestry is paramount. They become the guardian of your hopes and dreams, the compassionate companion who holds your hand through every twist and turn.

You find yourself in the midst of a heartfelt conversation with your healthcare provider. Their eyes sparkle with empathy and kindness, and their words resonate with understanding. They take the time to answer your questions, address your fears, and offer a gentle reassurance that no concern is too small. In their presence, you feel heard, valued, and empowered. This connection, grounded in trust and compassion, becomes the cornerstone of your prenatal care journey.

Together with your healthcare provider, you embark on a path of shared decision-making and open communication. They guide you through the maze of choices, from prenatal vitamins and nutrition to exercise and lifestyle adjustments. They educate you on the changes unfolding within your body, helping you embrace the physical and emotional transformations with grace and confidence.

You stand in front of a mirror, your hands gently caressing the gentle curve of your growing belly. You marvel at the miracle taking place within you, knowing that each stretch mark, each fluttering kick, is a testament to the life blossoming inside. And as you look deeper into your reflection, you recognize the strength and resilience that have awakened within you. It is the result of the unwavering support and guidance of your healthcare provider, who has instilled in you a profound belief in your ability to navigate the challenges and joys of motherhood.

Prenatal care extends beyond the realm of medical appointments. It is a holistic approach to nurturing your mind, body, and spirit. Your healthcare provider encourages you to embrace self-care practices that promote emotional well-being, such as mindfulness exercises, journaling, or seeking support from prenatal support groups. They remind you that taking care of yourself is not selfish but an essential part of nurturing your baby.

You find yourself sitting in a peaceful corner of your home, a soft blanket wrapped around your shoulders, a journal and pen in your hands. As you pour your thoughts onto the pages, emotions cascade like a gentle waterfall. You release your fears, celebrate your joys, and express your hopes for the future. In this intimate act of self-reflection, you realize that by caring for yourself, you are also caring for your baby. The love and nurturing you invest in your own well-being ripple outward, embracing the life within you.

Understanding the importance of prenatal care and selecting a healthcare provider who cherishes your journey is a profound and emotional endeavor. It is an affirmation of the boundless love and dedication you hold for your unborn child. Prenatal care becomes a tapestry of support, guidance, and empowerment, weaving together the threads of your maternal instincts and the expertise of your healthcare provider. It is a dance of vulnerability and strength, as you surrender to the awe-inspiring journey of creating life.

As you progress through your prenatal care, remember that you are not alone. Your healthcare provider is there to celebrate your triumphs, hold your hand during moments of uncertainty, and provide solace when the weight of responsibility feels overwhelming. They become your confidant, your cheerleader, and your guardian angel, offering a steadfast presence throughout the ebb and flow of your pregnancy.

It's a quiet evening, and you find yourself nestled in the comfort of your home, cradling your baby bump. The room is bathed in a warm glow, and a soft melody fills the air. You close your eyes and begin to visualize the support and love that surrounds you. In this moment, you feel the collective strength of your healthcare provider, your loved ones, and the countless mothers who have journeyed before you. It is a tapestry of shared experiences and shared wisdom, reminding you that you are part of a vast sisterhood of mothers.

As you navigate the labyrinth of prenatal care, remember that it is not merely a destination but a transformative journey. Each appointment, test, and conversation is an opportunity to deepen your connection with your baby, to unveil the miracles unfolding within you. It is a tapestry of moments—a tender heartbeat, a first flutter, a tiny hand waving on an ultrasound screen—that etch themselves into the fabric of your soul, forever shaping your identity as a mother.

You find yourself sitting in a waiting room, surrounded by expectant mothers with their own stories and dreams. As you share smiles and knowing glances, you realize the profound bond that unites you all. In that shared space, a sense of belonging blossoms—a recognition that you are part of a sacred tapestry of life, each thread intertwining to form the intricate pattern of motherhood.

In the midst of prenatal care, allow yourself to surrender to the waves of emotion that wash over you. Embrace the tears that flow, whether from joy, fear, or a beautiful mixture of both. These tears are the essence of your love, a tangible expression of the depths of your heart. They are a reminder that motherhood is not just about the physical journey of carrying a child, but an emotional odyssey that stretches and expands your capacity to love.

In the embrace of prenatal care, you will witness the miraculous growth of your baby, feel the rhythm of their life within you, and prepare yourself to welcome them into the world. It is a journey that will leave an indelible mark on your soul, forever changing you in ways you never thought possible.

Prenatal Check-ups and Test

Prenatal check-ups and tests play a crucial role in ensuring the health and well-being of both the expectant mother and the developing baby. Here are some professional tips on the importance of prenatal check-ups and tests:

1. **Early detection of potential issues:** Regular prenatal check-ups allow healthcare providers to monitor the progress of the pregnancy and detect any potential complications or health issues early on. This early detection can lead to timely interventions and better outcomes for both the mother and the baby.

2. **Monitoring the baby's growth and development:** Prenatal check-ups involve measurements of the baby's growth, such as fetal heart rate, size, and position. These assessments help healthcare providers ensure that the baby is growing properly and reaching important developmental milestones.

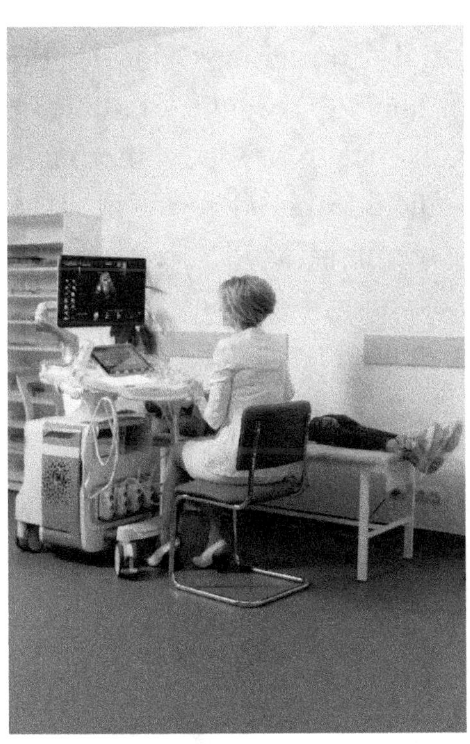

3. **Assessing maternal health:** Prenatal check-ups are not only focused on the baby but also on the

mother's health. These appointments allow healthcare providers to monitor the mother's blood pressure, weight, and overall well-being. They can identify any potential risks or complications that may arise during pregnancy and take appropriate measures to address them.

4. **Managing existing health conditions:** For women with pre-existing medical conditions, prenatal check-ups are essential for managing and monitoring those conditions throughout pregnancy. Healthcare providers can adjust treatment plans or provide specialized care to ensure both the mother and the baby are healthy.

5. **Providing essential screenings and tests:** Prenatal check-ups include a range of screenings and tests to assess the health of the mother and the baby. These may include blood tests, ultrasound scans, genetic screenings, and screenings for gestational diabetes and infections. These tests help identify any potential issues or risks and allow for appropriate management and intervention.

6. **Educating and counseling:** Prenatal check-ups offer an opportunity for healthcare providers to educate expectant mothers about pregnancy, childbirth, and postpartum care. They can address any concerns or questions the mother may have

and provide guidance on healthy lifestyle choices, nutrition, and preparation for childbirth.

7. **Establishing a trusting relationship:** Regular prenatal check-ups allow expectant mothers to develop a trusting relationship with their healthcare providers. This relationship is important for open communication, addressing concerns, and making informed decisions throughout the pregnancy journey.

8. **Emotional support:** Prenatal check-ups provide an avenue for emotional support. Pregnancy can bring about various emotions and concerns, and healthcare providers are there to offer guidance, reassurance, and a listening ear.

9. **Postpartum planning:** Prenatal check-ups also include discussions and planning for the postpartum period. This may involve preparing for breastfeeding, discussing contraception options, and addressing any concerns related to postpartum recovery and mental health.

10. **Continuity of care:** Regular prenatal check-ups ensure continuity of care throughout the pregnancy. They allow healthcare providers to monitor changes, provide appropriate interventions, and coordinate care with other specialists if necessary.

Choosing a Healthcare Provider

Choosing a healthcare provider who aligns with your birth preferences is an important decision that can greatly impact your pregnancy and childbirth experience. Here are some expert tips on how to select a healthcare provider who shares your birth philosophy:

1. **Do your research:** Start by researching different healthcare providers in your area and their approach to pregnancy and childbirth. Look for information on their website, online reviews, and social media. You can also ask for recommendations from family, friends, or a local childbirth education group.

2. **Consider their experience:** Look for healthcare providers with experience in the type of birth you want. For example, if you are considering a home birth, look for providers who have experience with home births. Ask about their qualifications, training, and experience with high-risk pregnancies or complications.

3. **Evaluate their communication style:** A good healthcare provider should be a good listener and communicator. During your initial consultation, pay attention to how they respond to your questions and concerns. Do they take the time to

explain things in a way that is easy to understand? Do they respect your preferences and values?

4. **Assess their approach to interventions:** If you have specific preferences regarding medical interventions during childbirth, ask about the provider's approach to interventions such as inductions, epidurals, or cesarean sections. Look for providers who support informed decision-making and provide options for natural childbirth.

5. **Consider their availability and accessibility:** It's important to choose a healthcare provider who is accessible and available to answer your questions and concerns. Ask about their availability for appointments, their response time to calls or messages, and their policy for after-hours emergencies.

6. **Evaluate their support team:** In addition to the healthcare provider, evaluate the support team they work with. This may include nurses, midwives, or doulas. Look for a team that shares your values and approach to childbirth.

7. **Trust your instincts:** Ultimately, the decision to choose a healthcare provider is a personal one. Listen to your instincts and choose a provider who makes you feel comfortable, supported, and empowered throughout your pregnancy and childbirth journey.

Choosing a healthcare provider who aligns with your birth preferences is an important step towards achieving the birth experience you desire. Take the time to research and evaluate your options, ask questions, and trust your instincts when making this decision.

Creating Birth Plans and Understanding Your Options

Creating a birth plan is an important step in preparing for childbirth. It helps you communicate your preferences and desires for your birth experience to your healthcare provider and support team. Here are some expert tips on creating a birth plan and understanding your options:

1. **Do your research:** Start by researching your options for childbirth. This may include different types of childbirth settings such as hospital, birth center, or home birth, as well as pain management options, labor and delivery positions, and interventions such as induction or cesarean section.

2. **Involve your healthcare provider:** Your healthcare provider can provide valuable guidance and support in creating your birth plan. Discuss your preferences and options with your provider, and ask for their input and recommendations.

3. **Keep it flexible:** While a birth plan can help you communicate your preferences, it's important to remember that childbirth can be unpredictable. Keep your plan flexible and be prepared to adjust as needed based on the needs of you and your baby.

4. **Communicate your preferences clearly:** Your birth plan should clearly communicate your preferences for your childbirth experience. Include information such as your desired pain management methods, labor and delivery positions, and preferences for interventions.

5. **Consider your support team:** Your support team can play an important role in helping you achieve the birth experience you desire. Consider including your partner, family members, or a doula in your birth plan and discuss their roles and responsibilities.

6. **Review your plan with your healthcare provider:** Once you have created your birth plan, review it with your healthcare provider to ensure that it aligns with their recommendations and the policies of your chosen childbirth setting.

7. **Be prepared to advocate for yourself:** While your healthcare provider and support team will work to support your preferences, it's important to be prepared to advocate for yourself and your

desires during childbirth. This may involve speaking up and asking questions, or seeking additional support or guidance.

Creating a birth plan can help you prepare for childbirth and communicate your preferences to your healthcare provider and support team. By doing your research, involving your healthcare provider, and keeping your plan flexible, you can help increase your chances of achieving the birth experience you desire.

So, dear mother-to-be, as you embark on this remarkable voyage of prenatal care, hold onto the profound emotions that accompany it. Cherish the connection with your healthcare provider, for they are the beacon of light guiding you through the vast expanse of pregnancy. Trust in the wisdom of your body, for it carries the essence of generations past and the promise of generations to come.

With each heartbeat, every kick, and the gentle whispers of your intuition, you will continue to prepare yourself—mind, body, and spirit—for the sacred role of motherhood. And as you do, remember that you are a vessel of love, chosen to nurture and protect the precious life growing within you. Embrace this emotional tapestry, for it is woven with the threads of unconditional love, resilience, and the awe-inspiring miracle of new beginnings.

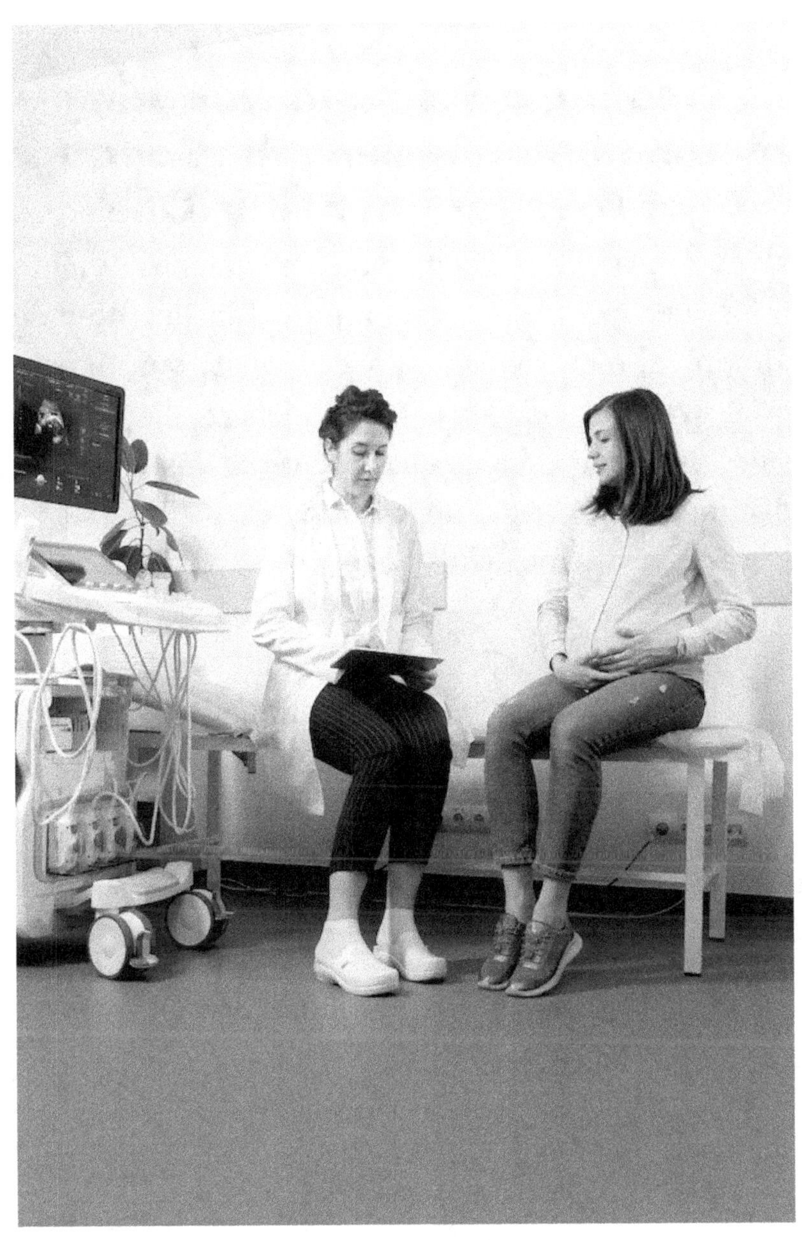

Chapter 4

Creating a Safe and Nurturing Environment: Unveiling the Sanctuary of Love for Your Little One

As you prepare to welcome your precious baby into the world, your heart brims with a primal instinct to protect and nurture. You envision a haven where your little one can thrive, a sanctuary of love where their laughter echoes and their dreams take flight. In this chapter, we delve into the profound importance of creating a safe and nurturing environment for your baby—one that will lay

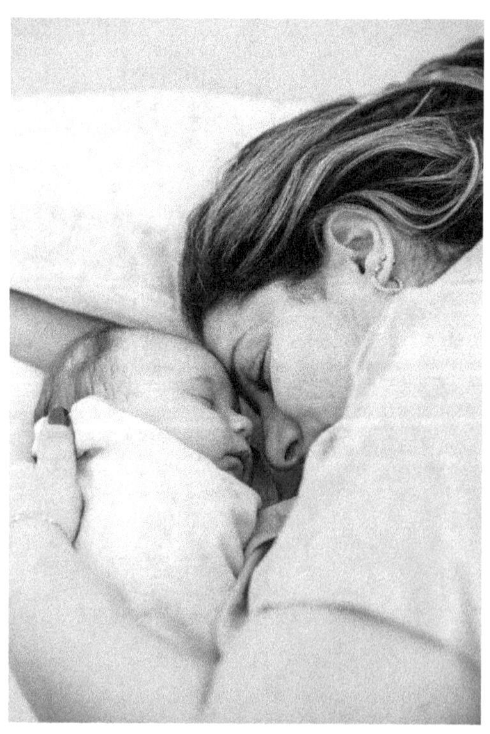

the foundation for their emotional well-being, growth, and flourishing. Let us embark on this emotional journey together as we unveil the sanctuary of love that awaits your little one.

You step into the nursery, the soft glow of the nightlight casting a gentle

53

luminescence. The room is adorned with tender touches—a cozy crib, a rocking chair for lullabies, and shelves filled with beloved books and toys. In this space, every detail has been thoughtfully chosen, emanating warmth and security. As you take in the scene, tears of anticipation and love blur your vision, for you know that this room holds the power to cradle your baby's dreams and cocoon them in a sense of belonging.

Creating a safe and nurturing environment for your baby goes beyond mere physical surroundings. It is a tapestry woven with emotional threads, encompassing love, empathy, and a deep understanding of your little one's needs. It is about creating an atmosphere where your baby feels seen, heard, and cherished—a space that becomes their sanctuary amidst the vastness of the world.

You cradle your newborn in your arms, their tiny fingers wrapped around yours. As you gaze into their eyes, you recognize the depth of trust that they place in you. In that tender moment, you make a vow—a sacred promise to create an environment where your baby will feel safe, loved, and valued. It is a pledge that will shape every decision you make as a parent, from the physical layout of their surroundings to the emotional presence you offer.

To create a safe and nurturing environment, start by addressing the physical aspects of your baby's surroundings. Ensure that their sleeping area is free from hazards, with a firm mattress, fitted sheets, and no loose blankets or pillows. Create a gentle ambiance through soft lighting, soothing colors, and calming scents. Remember, your baby's senses are delicate and attuned to the environment around them, so cultivate an atmosphere that embraces serenity and tranquility.

You hold your baby in your arms, the weight of their slumbering body a testament to their trust in your protection. You nestle them into a cozy swaddle, the fabric wrapping them in a warm embrace. As you softly hum a lullaby, the room transforms into a haven of tranquility. The soft glow of a nightlight casts a warm halo, and the subtle scent of lavender dances in the air. In this gentle cocoon, your baby drifts into a peaceful sleep, knowing they are cradled in your love.

Beyond the physical, the emotional climate you cultivate within your home plays a pivotal role in creating a safe and nurturing environment for your little one. Embrace the power of your presence—your voice, touch, and loving gaze. Engage in heartfelt conversations, even if your baby can't understand the words, for it is the tone and cadence of your voice that carries the resonance of love. Let your touch be a gentle caress, a soothing balm that calms their fears and imbues them with a sense of security.

You sit on the floor, surrounded by a flurry of toys and giggles. Your baby crawls towards you, their eyes shining with joy, and reaches out their arms. You open your arms, inviting them into a warm embrace. As you hold them close, you feel the rhythm of their breath, the beat of their heart against your chest. In this intimate connection, you communicate a language beyond words—the language of love and unconditional acceptance. Your touch becomes a symphony of reassurance, a testament to the safe haven you provide.

Creating a safe and nurturing environment also involves fostering a sense of routine and predictability. Babies thrive when they have a sense of structure and familiarity. Establish daily rituals that offer comfort and stability—a consistent bedtime routine, regular mealtimes, and moments of play and exploration. These routines become anchors in your baby's world, providing a sense of security amidst the ever-changing landscape of their early experiences.

It's bedtime, and you dim the lights in the nursery. As you follow the familiar steps of the bedtime routine—bathing, dressing, reading a bedtime story—you watch as your baby's eyes grow heavy with drowsiness. They snuggle into the softness of their blanket, finding solace in the familiarity of this nightly ritual. In these moments, you witness the power of routine, as it transforms the transition from wakefulness to sleep into a peaceful and comforting journey.

In creating a safe and nurturing environment, it is essential to cultivate a supportive network of loved ones. Surround yourself and your baby with individuals who share your values, respect your parenting choices, and offer unwavering support. Seek out community groups, parenting classes, or online forums where you can connect with other parents on a similar journey. The camaraderie and shared experiences provide a wellspring of emotional nourishment for both you and your baby.

Consider this relatable example: You gather with a group of fellow parents, the air buzzing with laughter and heartfelt conversations. As you exchange stories and advice, you realize that you are not alone in the challenges and joys of parenthood. In this community of shared experiences, you find solace, guidance, and a collective embrace that wraps around you and your baby. It is a reminder that you are part of something greater—a village of love and support.

Creating a safe and nurturing environment also involves being attuned to your baby's unique needs and cues. Pay close attention to their body language, facial expressions, and sounds. Learn to decipher their cries, understanding that each cry carries a message—a need for comfort, hunger, or connection. Respond to their cues promptly and tenderly, building a foundation of trust and emotional security.

Your baby's cry pierces the silence of the night, stirring you from sleep. You rush to their side, gathering them into your arms. As you hold them close, you soothe their tears with a gentle touch and a whispered lullaby. In that moment, you become attuned to their needs, recognizing that your response is more than just addressing their physical discomfort—it is a profound act of love and validation.

As you continue to create a safe and nurturing environment for your baby, remember to prioritize your own well-being. Self-care is not a luxury but a necessity, as it replenishes your emotional reserves, allowing you to show up fully for your little one. Take moments for yourself—whether it's a walk in nature, a warm bath, or simply a quiet moment of reflection. Nurture your own emotional well-being, for your baby's world is intricately connected to your own.

The soft glow of dawn filters through the curtains as you awaken to a new day. Before tending to your baby's needs, you take a few moments for yourself. You sit in a cozy corner, cradling a cup of tea, and bask in the quiet stillness. In this gentle pause, you nourish your own soul, replenishing the reservoir of love and strength within you. As you fill your cup, you are better equipped to pour love and care into your baby's world, creating a ripple effect of emotional well-being and nurturance.

Creating a safe and nurturing environment for your baby is a continuous journey—one that evolves as your little one grows and develops. Stay open to the ever-changing needs of your child, adjusting your approach with flexibility and compassion. Trust your instincts as a parent, for you possess an innate wisdom that guides you on this sacred path.

You watch in awe as your baby takes their first steps, their eyes shining with determination. As they navigate the world around them, you are reminded that creating a safe and nurturing environment is not confined to the physical space—it extends to the intangible realms of love, support, and encouragement. You become their biggest cheerleader, celebrating their milestones, soothing their falls, and fostering an environment where they feel brave to explore and grow.

In the tapestry of creating a safe and nurturing environment, remember that it is not about achieving perfection but embracing authenticity. Allow yourself the grace to make mistakes, for it is through imperfections that growth and connection flourish. Embrace vulnerability and transparency, sharing your joys and struggles with your little one. In doing so, you model resilience, empathy, and the beauty of embracing one's authentic self.

You sit with your toddler, flipping through the pages of a photo album filled with cherished memories. You share stories of their infancy, the triumphs and the challenges, the laughter and the tears. In this exchange, you create a sacred space where vulnerability is honored and connection deepens. Your child learns that their emotions and experiences are valid, and they are encouraged to navigate the complexities of life with courage and authenticity.

As you conclude this chapter, take a moment to envision the safe and nurturing environment you are creating for your baby. Picture their radiant smile, their eyes filled with trust and love. Know that your efforts, fueled by an immeasurable love, are shaping the very foundation of their well-being. Your commitment to providing a sanctuary of love will echo throughout their lives, fostering resilience, self-worth, and the capacity to love and be loved.

In the sanctuary of your love, your baby will blossom and flourish. They will take their first steps, explore their passions, and embark on their own journey of self-discovery. And as they grow, they will carry the indelible imprint of your safe and nurturing environment—a sanctuary that forever remains etched in their hearts and guides them as they navigate the vast tapestry of life.

Preparing Your Home for the Arrival of Your Baby

Preparing your home for the arrival of your baby is an exciting and important task. Here are some expert tips on how to get your home ready:

1. **Create a safe environment:** Ensure that your home is a safe place for your baby. Install safety gates at the top and bottom of stairs, secure heavy furniture to the wall to prevent tipping, cover electrical outlets, and use corner protectors on sharp edges. Remove any small objects or choking hazards from accessible areas.

2. **Set up the nursery:** Prepare a cozy and functional nursery for your baby. Choose a crib or bassinet that meets safety standards and position it away from cords, windows, and heavy objects. Set up a changing station with diapers, wipes, and diaper rash cream. Organize baby essentials, such as clothing, blankets, and burp cloths, for easy access.

3. **Stock up on baby supplies:** Ensure you have an ample supply of diapers, wipes, formula (if

applicable), and other baby essentials. Consider purchasing a baby monitor to keep an eye on your little one, and have a well-stocked first aid kit with items such as a thermometer, nasal aspirator, and infant-safe medication.

4. **Prepare feeding areas:** If you plan to breastfeed, create a comfortable and private area in your home for nursing. Consider investing in a comfortable nursing chair or pillow. If bottle-feeding, ensure you have sterilized bottles, nipples, and formula preparation supplies.

5. **Babyproof the common areas:** Assess the common areas of your home and take necessary babyproofing measures. Install safety latches on cabinets, secure loose cords, and remove fragile or hazardous items from low shelves or tables. Anchor heavy furniture that could pose a tipping risk.

6. **Stock your pantry:** As you adjust to life with a newborn, having easily accessible snacks and meals is essential. Stock your pantry with nutritious, ready-to-eat options, such as granola bars, nuts, and dried fruits. Consider prepping some freezer meals or arranging for meal deliveries during the early days.

7. **Prepare a diaper changing station:** Create a convenient diaper changing station in multiple

areas of your home. Stock it with diapers, wipes, diaper cream, and a changing pad. Having these essentials within reach can make diaper changes quicker and more efficient.

8. **Establish a laundry routine:** Babies generate a lot of laundry, so establish a laundry routine that works for you. Make sure you have a sufficient supply of baby-friendly laundry detergent and consider organizing your baby's clothes and linens with labeled storage bins or drawers.

9. **Create a calming atmosphere:** Consider creating a soothing and calming atmosphere in your home. Use soft lighting, play soothing music, and consider introducing items like a white noise machine or a baby swing to help comfort and relax your baby.

10. **Seek support:** Reach out to family, friends, or support groups for help and guidance as you prepare your home for your baby's arrival. Accepting assistance with organizing, cleaning, or setting up can alleviate some of the stress and allow you to focus on bonding with your newborn.

Preparing your home for your baby's arrival can help create a safe and nurturing environment. By following these expert tips, you can ensure that your home is ready to welcome your little one and support your transition into parenthood.

Babyproofing Your Home

Babyproofing your home is essential to create a safe environment for your little one as they explore and grow. Here are some expert tips on babyproofing essentials and safety guidelines:

1.   **Secure electrical outlets and cords:** Cover all electrical outlets with outlet covers or safety plugs to prevent your baby from sticking their fingers or objects into them. Additionally, secure cords and wires out of reach or use cord covers to eliminate potential hazards.

2.   **Install safety gates:** Place safety gates at the top and bottom of staircases, as well as in doorways to rooms or areas that you want to keep off-limits to your baby. Choose gates that are sturdy, properly installed, and meet safety standards.

3.   **Anchor furniture and appliances:** Secure heavy furniture, such as bookshelves, dressers, and TVs, to the wall to prevent tipping. Use furniture anchors or wall brackets to ensure stability and reduce the risk of accidents.

4.   **Lock cabinets and drawers:** Use childproof locks or safety latches on cabinets and drawers within your baby's reach. This prevents them from accessing potentially harmful items like cleaning supplies, sharp objects, or medications.

5.   **Cover sharp corners and edges:** Apply corner guards or cushioned edge protectors to sharp corners and edges of furniture or countertops to minimize the risk of injury if your baby falls or bumps into them.

6.   **Keep small objects out of reach:** Remove small objects, such as coins, buttons, or small toys, from areas where your baby can reach them. These items can pose a choking hazard.

7.   **Use window safety measures:** Install window guards or window stops to prevent your baby from falling out of windows. Ensure that window blind cords are kept out of reach or use cordless blinds to eliminate the risk of strangulation.

8.   **Install toilet locks:** Use toilet locks to prevent your baby from accessing the toilet bowl, which can be a drowning hazard. Keep bathroom doors closed and consider using non-slip mats in the bathtub to prevent slips and falls.

9.   **Secure heavy appliances:** Ensure that heavy appliances, such as ovens and dishwashers, are

properly secured to prevent tipping or accidental injury.

10.   **Monitor water temperature:** Adjust your water heater to a safe temperature to prevent scalding. Test the water temperature before bathing your baby using a bath thermometer or by checking with your elbow or wrist.

11.   **Cover unused electrical outlets:** For outlets not in use, use outlet covers or safety plugs to prevent your baby from inserting objects into them.

12.**Be cautious with cords and blinds:** Keep blind cords and curtain strings out of reach or use cord wraps or cordless options to avoid strangulation hazards.

13.**Securely close doors and gates:** Install doorstops or door holders to prevent your baby's fingers from getting pinched or slammed in doors. Be mindful of hinges and ensure they are not a risk to your baby's tiny fingers.

14. **Supervise your baby:** While babyproofing is important, it's crucial to remember that supervision is the most effective safety measure. Keep a watchful eye on your baby at all times, especially when they are in new environments or around potential hazards.

Babyproofing is an ongoing process as your baby grows and develops new abilities. Regularly reassess your home for potential hazards and make necessary adjustments to ensure a safe environment for your little one.

Designing a Cozy Nursery for Your Little One

Designing a cozy nursery for your little one is an exciting and creative process. Here are some tips to help you create a warm and inviting space for your baby:

1. **Choose soothing colors:** Opt for soft, calming colors such as pastels, neutrals, or gentle shades of blue or pink. These colors create a serene atmosphere that promotes relaxation and sleep.
2. **Consider the lighting:** Use a combination of natural and artificial lighting to create a cozy ambiance. Install blackout curtains or blinds to control the amount of light coming in during nap times. Use a dimmable overhead light and incorporate soft, warm lighting with table lamps or nightlights for a soothing glow.
3. **Select comfortable furniture:** Invest in a comfortable crib or bassinet with a quality mattress that meets safety standards. Choose a glider or rocking chair with plush cushions where you can comfortably nurse, cuddle, or read to your baby.

Add a side table or shelf to keep essentials within reach.

4. **Create a functional layout:** Arrange the furniture in a way that allows for easy movement and accessibility. Place the crib in a central location and ensure there is ample space for walking around and attending to your baby's needs.

5. **Incorporate soft textures:** Use soft, cozy textiles to add warmth and comfort to the nursery. Consider using plush rugs, soft blankets, and pillows. Opt for curtains or drapes made from gentle fabrics to create a soft, dreamy atmosphere.

6. **Personalize the space:** Add personal touches to make the nursery feel special and unique. Hang artwork, framed photos, or a personalized name sign. Consider adding a growth chart or a memory board where you can showcase milestones and memories.

7. **Organize storage solutions:** Incorporate practical storage solutions to keep the nursery organized and clutter-free. Use baskets, bins, or shelves to store diapers, wipes, clothing, toys, and other baby essentials. A well-organized space promotes a sense of calm and makes it easier to find what you need.

8. **Consider a theme or style:** Choose a theme or style that resonates with you and creates a cozy

atmosphere. It can be based on a favorite animal, nature, a storybook, or a specific color palette. Incorporate elements that reflect the theme through wall decals, bedding, or artwork.

9. **Add soft sounds and music:** Consider playing soft, soothing music or white noise in the nursery. Gentle melodies or calming sounds can create a peaceful environment that promotes relaxation and helps your baby settle down.

10. **Ensure a safe environment:** As you design the nursery, prioritize safety. Follow safety guidelines for crib placement, secure furniture to the wall to prevent tipping, ensure cords and wires are out of reach, and use childproofing measures on outlets and drawers.

The most important aspect of a cozy nursery is the love and care you provide to your little one. Design a space that reflects your style and preferences while prioritizing comfort, safety, and functionality. Enjoy the process and create a nurturing environment where you and your baby can bond and create beautiful memories.

Dear parent, embrace the sacred responsibility bestowed upon you. Embrace the power of your love, the depth of your intuition, and the transformative role you play in shaping your baby's world. Through your unwavering commitment to creating a safe and nurturing environment, you gift your little one with the greatest treasure of all—the unwavering assurance that they are loved, cherished, and protected.

Chapter 5

Building a Supportive Network: Weaving Threads of Love and Connection

In the beautiful tapestry of parenthood, there are moments of immense joy, boundless love, and awe-inspiring growth. Yet, there are also challenges, uncertainties, and moments when you may feel overwhelmed. In these times, having a supportive network can make all the difference—a constellation of loving souls who embrace you, lift you up, and share in the triumphs and trials of your journey. This chapter explores the profound importance of building a supportive network as you navigate the transformative path of parenthood, weaving threads of love and connection that will sustain and nourish you along the way.

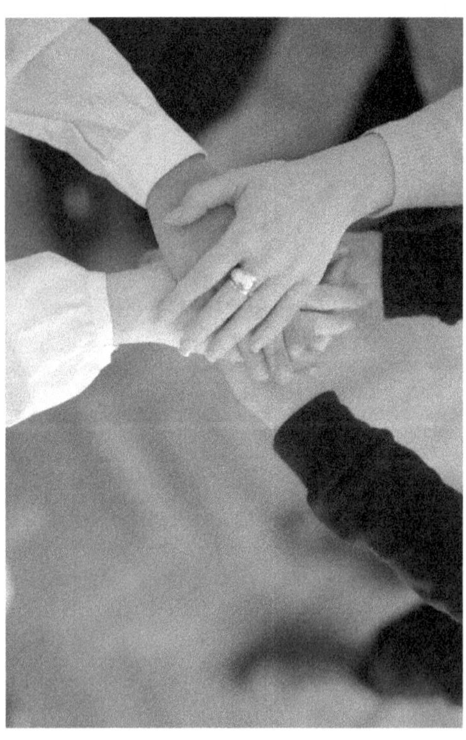

You hold your baby close, their tiny hand

wrapped around your finger. In that tender embrace, you realize that you are embarking on a journey that is both miraculous and humbling. Parenthood is a transformative experience that stretches the boundaries of your heart, and it is in these moments that the support of others becomes invaluable. As you gaze into your baby's eyes, you recognize the importance of building a network of love and support—a safety net that will catch you when you stumble, lift you when you fall, and celebrate with you when you soar.

Building a supportive network starts with reaching out to your loved ones—family, friends, and those who have walked the path of parenthood before you. **Share your hopes, fears, and dreams with them.** Open your heart and vulnerability, allowing them to witness your journey and offer their unwavering support. You will be amazed by the love and wisdom they bring, as their experiences become guiding lights in your own parenthood adventure.

You gather with your closest friends and family, your living room alive with laughter and joy. As you share the news of your impending arrival, you are met with an outpouring of love, excitement, and congratulations. In that moment, you realize that you are not alone in this journey. Your loved ones become the pillars of your support network, ready to lend an ear, offer advice, and shower your little one with affection. Their presence weaves a thread of connection that strengthens the foundation of your growing family.

Beyond your immediate circle, seek out communities of like-minded parents who can offer guidance, empathy, and shared experiences. Join parenting groups, attend support classes, or connect with online communities. These spaces provide fertile ground for cultivating connections with individuals who understand the unique challenges and joys of parenthood. Together, you form a tribe—a collective web of support that embraces you in times of need and celebrates your triumphs.

You attend a parenting class, surrounded by other expectant mothers and fathers. The room buzzes with anticipation and curiosity. As you exchange stories and tips, you discover a shared bond that transcends age, background, and experience. In this circle of understanding, you find solace, guidance, and an unwavering support system that accompanies you on your parenting journey. The relationships formed in these spaces become lifelines that sustain you through the highs and lows of parenthood.

Building a supportive network also involves seeking professional support when needed. Reach out to healthcare providers, lactation consultants, therapists, and other experts who can offer guidance and expertise. These individuals play a crucial role in your journey, providing reassurance, medical advice, and the tools to navigate the complexities of parenthood. They become trusted allies who stand beside you, ensuring the well-being of both you and your baby.

You sit in the office of a lactation consultant, feeling a mix of exhaustion and determination. As you share your breastfeeding challenges, the consultant listens attentively, offering practical strategies and words of encouragement. In that moment, a weight lifts off your shoulders. **You realize that you are not alone in your struggles.** The lactation consultant becomes a guiding light, providing you with the tools and knowledge to overcome obstacles and nourish your baby with love and care. Their expertise and unwavering support become instrumental in your breastfeeding journey, reminding you that you are capable and deserving of success.

Building a supportive network also means finding your tribe of fellow parents who are walking a similar path. Seek out parent support groups, both in-person and online, where you can connect with others who share similar values and parenting philosophies. These groups provide a safe space to share experiences, exchange advice, and offer a listening ear during the moments of doubt and uncertainty.

You attend a local parent support group, filled with mothers and fathers who gather to share their stories. As you sit in a circle, passing around tissues and laughter, you realize the power of this collective.

In this space, you find validation and understanding as others nod in empathy and share their own struggles and triumphs. You form deep connections, knowing that these individuals will be there to cheer you on and lift you up during the challenges that lie ahead. Building a supportive network also extends beyond the realm of parenthood. Nurture your friendships, even as life takes on a new dimension with the arrival of your baby. Lean on trusted friends who have been by your side through thick and thin. These friends, who have witnessed your journey long before parenthood, offer a sense of continuity and familiarity. They remind you of your identity beyond being a parent, honoring and celebrating all aspects of who you are.

You gather with your closest friends for an evening of laughter and connection. As you share stories and reminisce about old times, you realize the importance of preserving these relationships amidst the whirlwind of parenthood. Your friends become the guardians of your spirit, reminding you of the person you were before becoming a parent and loving you unconditionally in your new role. Their presence becomes a sanctuary, a space where you can rejuvenate and find solace amidst the beautiful chaos of parenting.

Building a supportive network is not only about receiving support but also about giving it. Be present for your loved ones, offering a listening ear, words of encouragement, and a helping hand whenever needed. Celebrate their milestones and victories, just as they celebrate yours. In the tapestry of relationships, the threads of love and support are interwoven, creating a web of interconnectedness that sustains and nourishes all who are a part of it.

Your friend, also a new parent, reaches out to you in the midst of a sleepless night. They are exhausted and overwhelmed, seeking reassurance and guidance. In that moment, you hold space for them, offering a shoulder to lean on and words of empathy. Your presence becomes a source of strength, reminding them that they are not alone in their struggles. Through your support, you become an integral part of their network, weaving threads of love and connection that withstand the tests of time.

In the tapestry of parenthood, building a supportive network is an essential component—a lifeline that sustains you during the moments of doubt, fatigue, and uncertainty. It is a testament to the power of human connection and the profound impact it has on our well-being and growth. Embrace the opportunity to weave threads of love and support, for in doing so, you create a safety net that will carry you through the peaks and valleys of your parenting journey.

As you continue to weave the tapestry of your parenting journey, remember that building a supportive network is not solely about seeking assistance during challenging times. It is also about nurturing and cherishing the connections that uplift your spirit, ignite your joy, and celebrate the milestones and precious moments of your little one's life.

It's a sunny afternoon, and you gather with your newfound parent friends in a local park. The laughter of children fills the air as your little ones explore the world together. As you sit on a blanket, sharing stories and trading parenting tips, you realize the immense beauty of these connections. In this circle of friendship, you find solace, inspiration, and a deep sense of belonging. The shared laughter, tears, and triumphs become the fabric that strengthens the bonds of your support network.

Within your supportive network, you may also find mentors—seasoned parents who have traversed the path before you and offer wisdom and guidance. Their experience becomes a beacon of hope and a source of inspiration, reassuring you that the challenges you face are part of the universal journey of parenthood. They share insights, offer advice, and lend a compassionate ear, reminding you that you are never alone in your struggles or triumphs.

You connect with a seasoned mother at a community gathering. As you share your concerns and uncertainties, she listens with empathy and kindness. She shares her own experiences, offering valuable lessons and practical suggestions. In that exchange, you discover the power of intergenerational support—a connection that spans generations and carries the wisdom of those who have walked this path before you. Her presence becomes a guiding light, illuminating your way and instilling you with the confidence to navigate the challenges of parenthood.

Building a supportive network also means embracing vulnerability—the willingness to ask for help and share your struggles openly. Recognize that reaching out does not diminish your strength as a parent; it magnifies it. It takes courage to acknowledge that you cannot do it all alone and to lean on others for support. By allowing yourself to be vulnerable, you create space for deep connections, compassion, and understanding to flourish.

Late at night, you find yourself overwhelmed with fatigue and the weight of responsibility. Tears stream down your face as you cradle your baby, feeling a mix of exhaustion and doubt. In that moment, you reach out to a trusted friend, sharing your raw emotions and fears. Their response is one of love and reassurance. They remind you of your resilience and offer their unwavering support. In this vulnerable exchange, you experience the power of genuine connection—the knowledge that you are seen, heard, and loved unconditionally.

As you build your supportive network, remember that it is a reciprocal relationship—a tapestry woven with threads of love, compassion, and reciprocity. Just as you receive support, be a source of strength and encouragement for others. Offer a listening ear, lend a helping hand, and celebrate the victories and joys of those around you. In doing so, you create a community that thrives on empathy, kindness, and shared experiences.

You attend a baby shower for a close friend, filled with excitement and anticipation. As you gather with others, you bring a gift not only for the baby but also a heartfelt note of encouragement and support for the new parents. In that moment, you embody the spirit of a supportive network, showering them with love and reminding them that they are not alone on this extraordinary journey. Your gesture of thoughtfulness becomes a thread in their tapestry, weaving connections that will endure beyond the baby shower.

In the tapestry of parenthood, building a supportive network is a testament to the beauty of human connection. It is a reminder that we are not alone in our struggles or joys. It is a recognition that we are all woven together in the intricate fabric of life, and through our connections, we find strength, resilience, and the capacity to thrive.

In the depths of the night, when exhaustion threatens to consume you, or when doubt creeps in during moments of uncertainty, your supportive network stands as a beacon of light, guiding you back to your own inner strength. Their presence reminds you that you are part of something greater—a community of love and understanding that stretches beyond time and space.

It's a rainy day, and you find yourself overwhelmed by the demands of parenting. The responsibilities pile up, and you feel like you're barely keeping your head above water. In that moment, you receive a message from a fellow parent in your support group. They offer words of encouragement, reminding you that the storm will pass and that you have what it takes to weather it. Their kindness and understanding warm your heart, reigniting your determination to carry on.

Within your supportive network, you may also find unexpected connections and friendships that transcend traditional boundaries. The bonds formed in this shared journey of parenthood are often profound, breaking down barriers and bringing people together who may have otherwise never crossed paths. Different backgrounds, cultures, and experiences merge into a tapestry of diversity and unity, enriching the fabric of your support network.

You attend a multicultural parenting group, where parents from various backgrounds gather to share their experiences. As you listen to stories of traditions, customs, and parenting practices, you realize the power of diversity in fostering understanding and growth. In this tapestry of cultures, you find inspiration and learn valuable lessons that shape your own parenting approach. The connections you form in this diverse community become a source of enrichment and broaden your perspective on what it means to be a parent.

As you navigate the ever-changing landscape of parenthood, your support network becomes a lifeline during times of transition and adjustment. They stand by your side, offering guidance and reassurance as you navigate the challenges of sleepless nights, developmental milestones, and the constant ebb and flow of your child's growth. Through their presence, you gain the strength to face each new phase with resilience and hope.

Your child is about to start preschool, and you find yourself filled with a mix of excitement and anxiety. In this moment of transition, you turn to your support network for guidance and encouragement. They share their own experiences, offering practical advice and a listening ear. Their reassurance helps ease your worries, allowing you to embrace this new chapter with confidence and optimism. Together, you navigate the path of parenthood, united in your commitment to the well-being and happiness of your children.

In the tapestry of parenthood, building a supportive network is not merely an option—it is an essential thread that weaves its way through the fabric of your journey. It is a tapestry that embraces vulnerability, fosters growth, and celebrates the shared experiences of parenthood. Through the strength of your connections, you find solace in the knowledge that you are never alone, that there are others who stand ready to offer their love, support, and understanding.

So, reach out and embrace the power of connection. Seek out those who share your joys, fears, and dreams. Build a supportive network that lifts you up, cheers you on, and holds you tight during the storms. For in the embrace of your community, you will find the courage, resilience, and love needed to navigate the intricate tapestry of parenthood. And as you weave your own thread into the lives of others, remember that your presence and support have the power to change lives and create a ripple effect of love and compassion that extends far beyond the boundaries of parenthood.

It's a bright summer day, and you gather with your support network at a local park. The laughter of children fills the air, intermingling with the sound of heartfelt conversations. As you sit on a blanket, surrounded by your trusted friends, you realize the immense power of this community. Each person brings their unique story, their own fears and hopes, and together, you form a tapestry of love and understanding. In this safe haven, you feel embraced, cherished, and seen for who you truly are—an incredible parent navigating the beautiful, messy, and extraordinary journey of raising a child.

Within your supportive network, you discover that the ties that bind you together go beyond shared experiences of parenthood. They are the friends who lend a helping hand when your spirit feels weary, who offer solace and comfort during moments of doubt, and who celebrate the smallest victories as if they were their own. Their unwavering presence becomes a testament to the beauty of human connection, reminding you that you are never alone on this path.

As you face the challenges of the early weeks of parenting, you reach out to a close friend who has become an integral part of your support network.

They arrive at your doorstep with a warm meal, a caring smile, and a listening ear. In that moment, their gesture of kindness fills your heart with gratitude and reminds you of the profound impact a supportive network can have on your well-being. Their presence becomes a lifeline, offering you a brief respite from the demands of parenthood and reaffirming that you are surrounded by love and support.

Building a supportive network also means embracing the vulnerability to share your deepest fears, insecurities, and joys. It is within these moments of authenticity that true connections are forged, as others recognize and validate your experiences. Through their empathy, they lift the weight off your shoulders, helping you find solace and strength in the shared human experience.

In a quiet corner of a coffee shop, you sit with a fellow parent from your support group. As you open up about the challenges and triumphs of your parenting journey, tears well up in your eyes. In that vulnerable exchange, your friend reaches across the table and grasps your hand. Their understanding gaze and gentle squeeze offer an unspoken affirmation of your worth as a parent. It is in these moments of raw authenticity that the bonds of friendship deepen, and you realize the transformative power of a supportive network.

Building a supportive network also extends beyond the boundaries of physical proximity. In today's interconnected world, technology allows us to forge meaningful connections with like-minded parents across the globe. Online communities, social media groups, and parenting forums become virtual sanctuaries where you can seek advice, share experiences, and find solace in the late hours of the night when the rest of the world is asleep.

In the dim glow of your phone screen, you scroll through a parenting forum, searching for answers to a burning question that keeps you awake at night. As you navigate through the threads, you stumble upon a post that resonates deeply with your own experience. In that virtual space, you find comfort in the shared struggles and triumphs of parents who understand your journey. The supportive comments and words of encouragement become a lifeline, reminding you that there is a vast community of kindred spirits who are only a click away.

In the tapestry of parenthood, building a supportive network becomes an essential part of your self-care. It is a testament to the resilience of the human spirit and the boundless capacity for love and connection. Through the web of relationships you create, you find solace, wisdom, and the courage to face the challenges that come your way. Embrace the intricate threads of your supportive network, for they are woven with love, compassion, and understanding.

Within your network, you may find a fellow parent who becomes your confidant, a pillar of strength during the darkest moments. They listen intently as you pour out your heart, sharing your deepest fears, insecurities, and the weight of your responsibilities. Their unwavering support and empathy provide a safe space for you to be vulnerable, offering a healing balm for your weary soul. In their presence, you feel validated, understood, and reminded that your struggles are not in vain.

It's a quiet evening, and you find yourself overwhelmed by the challenges of parenting. Emotions bubble up within you, threatening to engulf your spirit. In that moment, you reach out to your trusted friend—a fellow parent who has walked this path alongside you. They hold your hand, offering a listening ear and a compassionate heart. As you share your burdens, tears flow freely, releasing the pent-up emotions that have weighed you down. Their unwavering support and understanding bring a sense of relief and renewal, rekindling the flame of hope within you.

Building a supportive network also means celebrating the milestones, joys, and victories, both big and small, that mark your journey as a parent. Your network becomes a chorus of cheerleaders, rejoicing in your child's first steps, beaming with pride at their achievements, and sharing in the delight of every toothless grin and belly laugh. Their enthusiasm and shared joy amplify your own, creating an atmosphere of celebration that adds color and vibrancy to your parenting experience.

It's a sunny afternoon, and you attend a birthday party for your friend's child. As you gather with your supportive network, you witness the pure, unadulterated joy radiating from the little ones running around. Each milestone, from blowing out the candles on the cake to opening presents, is met with a chorus of cheers and applause. In that moment, you realize the power of a community that celebrates together—the contagious laughter, the gleeful smiles, and the shared sense of wonder. The energy of celebration infuses your spirit, reminding you of the beauty and magic inherent in the everyday moments of parenthood.

Building a supportive network also means embracing diversity and inclusivity. It is a tapestry that encompasses individuals from various backgrounds, cultures, and perspectives. These differences enrich your experience, expanding your horizons and challenging your preconceived notions. Within this mosaic of voices, you discover the power of collective wisdom—the collective wisdom that arises when individuals come together, united by a common purpose: to nurture and raise their children with love and compassion.

You attend a gathering of parents from diverse cultural backgrounds. The room is filled with the aroma of different cuisines, the sounds of languages intertwining, and the vibrant colors of traditional garments. As you engage in conversations and share stories, you are exposed to a tapestry of traditions, customs, and parenting practices. The exchange of knowledge, the curiosity to learn from one another, and the mutual respect that permeates the room create an atmosphere of unity and understanding. In this moment, you realize that your support network is not only a source of comfort and encouragement but also an opportunity for growth and cultural appreciation.

The Power of a Strong Support System

Recognizing the power of a strong support system is crucial, especially during the journey of parenthood. Here are some key points to understand the importance and benefits of having a strong support system:

1. **Emotional support:** A strong support system provides emotional encouragement, understanding, and empathy. They offer a listening ear when you need to express your joys, concerns, or challenges. Sharing your experiences and emotions with supportive individuals can help alleviate stress and provide a sense of comfort and validation.

2. **Practical assistance:** A support system can offer practical help when you need it the most. They can assist with tasks such as meal preparation, running errands, or providing childcare, giving you the opportunity to focus on your own well-being and the care of your baby.

3. **Knowledge and experience sharing:** Having a support system allows you to tap into the knowledge and experiences of others who have been through similar situations. They can provide advice, suggestions, and helpful tips based on their own parenting journeys. This collective wisdom can be invaluable in navigating the challenges and uncertainties of parenthood.

4. **Reduced feelings of isolation:** Parenthood can sometimes feel isolating, especially during periods of sleep deprivation, adjustment to new routines, or when facing unexpected difficulties. A strong support system helps combat feelings of loneliness by providing a sense of belonging and a network of individuals who understand and share your experiences.

5. **Increased self-care opportunities:** With a support system in place, you are more likely to have opportunities for self-care. Whether it's having someone to watch your baby while you take a break, or simply offering encouragement to prioritize your own well-being, a support system can help ensure that you have time to recharge and care for yourself.

6. **Enhanced problem-solving capabilities:** When faced with challenges or decisions, having a support system allows you to benefit from multiple perspectives. They can offer different insights and viewpoints, helping you explore various options and make informed decisions that align with your values and goals.

7. **Celebration of milestones:** A support system provides a group of individuals who will cheer on your baby's milestones and accomplishments. Whether it's a first smile, first steps, or any other

significant achievement, having a supportive network to share these moments with enhances the joy and pride of parenthood.

8. **Relieving stress and promoting mental well-being:** Research has shown that having a strong support system can reduce stress levels and promote better mental health. Having people who understand and genuinely care about your well-being can provide a sense of security and help you navigate the challenges of parenthood with greater ease.

Building a support system may involve reaching out to family members, friends, parenting groups, or online communities. It's essential to surround yourself with individuals who are positive, understanding, and supportive of your choices and parenting style.

Recognizing the power of a strong support system is a valuable aspect of parenthood. It not only benefits you but also creates a nurturing environment for your baby. Don't hesitate to lean on your support system and cultivate those connections, as they can play a significant role in your parenting journey.

Nurturing Relationships

Nurturing relationships with your partner, family, and friends is vital during the journey of parenthood. Here are some key points to consider when it comes to fostering and strengthening these important relationships:

1. **Open communication:** Maintain open and honest communication with your partner, family members, and friends. Share your thoughts, feelings, and concerns, and encourage them to do the same. Effective communication fosters understanding, resolves conflicts, and strengthens bonds.

2. **Quality time together:** Prioritize spending quality time with your partner, family, and friends. Set aside dedicated moments to connect and engage in activities that bring you joy and strengthen your relationships. It can be as simple as having a meal together, going for a walk, or enjoying a shared hobby.

3. **Express appreciation and gratitude:** Show appreciation and gratitude for the support, love, and involvement of your partner, family, and friends. Expressing gratitude not only nurtures the relationship but also fosters a positive and supportive atmosphere.

4. **Seek and offer support:** Be proactive in seeking support from your partner, family, and friends when needed. Similarly, be willing to provide support and assistance to them. By offering help and being there for one another, you create a sense of reciprocity and deepen your connections.

5. **Delegate responsibilities:** Share parenting responsibilities with your partner and involve other family members and friends whenever possible. Delegating tasks can help alleviate stress, create a sense of shared responsibility, and allow for more quality time together.

6. **Maintain individual connections:** While your focus may naturally shift to your baby, it's important to maintain individual connections with your partner, family members, and friends. Nurture these relationships by regularly checking in, scheduling one-on-one time, and showing genuine interest in their lives and well-being.

7. **Seek professional help if needed:** Sometimes, the challenges of parenthood can put a strain on relationships. If you find yourself facing significant difficulties, consider seeking professional help through couples therapy or counseling. These resources can provide guidance and support in navigating relationship challenges and strengthening bonds.

8. **Be flexible and understanding:** Understand that the dynamics of relationships may change as you navigate parenthood. Be flexible and adapt to the evolving needs and priorities of your partner, family,

and friends. Show empathy and understanding during this transitional period, and be patient with one another.

9. **Celebrate milestones together:** Include your partner, family, and friends in celebrating your baby's milestones. Share the joy and excitement of first words, steps, birthdays, and other significant moments. Involving loved ones creates a sense of shared happiness and strengthens the bond between them and your child.

10. **Practice self-care:** Taking care of yourself is essential in nurturing relationships. Prioritize self-care to maintain your well-being and emotional balance. When you prioritize your own needs, you can show up as a happier and more present partner, family member, and friend.

Nurturing relationships with your partner, family, and friends requires effort, time, and ongoing commitment. By investing in these connections, you create a strong support system that enhances your well-being and enriches your parenting journey. Remember that the bonds you foster will not only benefit you but also contribute to a nurturing and loving environment for your baby.

Connecting with Other Expectant Mom

Connecting with other expectant mothers and joining support groups can be a valuable part of your journey through pregnancy and motherhood. Here are some key points to consider when it comes to connecting with other expectant mothers and joining support groups:

1. **Seek out prenatal classes and workshops:** Look for prenatal classes or workshops in your community or online that bring together expectant mothers. These classes often provide a supportive environment where you can connect with other moms-to-be who are going through similar experiences. It's an opportunity to learn from experts, ask questions, and build relationships.

2. **Join online communities and forums:** There are numerous online communities and forums dedicated to expectant mothers. Joining these groups allows you to connect with women from around the world who are at various stages of pregnancy. These platforms provide a space for sharing stories, asking questions, and offering support. It can be a great way to find advice, recommendations, and emotional encouragement.

3. **Attend prenatal support groups:** Look for local prenatal support groups facilitated by professionals or organizations that focus on providing support for expectant mothers. These groups typically meet

regularly and offer a safe space to discuss concerns, share experiences, and receive guidance. Connecting with other expectant mothers in person can provide a sense of community and understanding.

4. **Utilize social media platforms:** Social media platforms, such as Facebook groups or Instagram communities, often have dedicated spaces for expectant mothers. These groups allow you to connect with like-minded individuals, share resources, and engage in discussions. It's important to find supportive and positive communities where you feel comfortable and can foster meaningful connections.

5. **Attend local events and meetups:** Keep an eye out for local events or meetups specifically designed for expectant mothers. These could include prenatal fitness classes, baby expos, or parenting workshops. Attending these events gives you the opportunity to meet other expectant mothers in your area and build relationships that can extend beyond pregnancy.

6. **Be open and approachable:** When interacting with other expectant mothers, be open and approachable. Initiate conversations, listen actively, and offer support. By creating a welcoming and inclusive environment, you

encourage others to share their experiences and build connections.

7. **Share your own journey:** As you connect with other expectant mothers, share your own experiences and insights. Your unique perspective may offer comfort or guidance to someone else. Sharing stories, tips, and resources creates a sense of camaraderie and fosters a supportive network.

8. **Attend childbirth education classes:** Consider enrolling in childbirth education classes with your partner. These classes often bring together couples who are preparing for the arrival of their babies. Connecting with other expectant parents can be an enriching experience and a way to establish friendships that may extend into the postpartum period.

9. **Be respectful of diverse experiences:** Remember that every expectant mothers journey is unique, and experiences can vary widely. Show respect for different perspectives and avoid judgment or comparison. Embrace the diversity within the group and foster an environment of empathy and understanding.

Connecting with other expectant mothers and joining support groups can provide a valuable network of support, guidance, and friendship during pregnancy and beyond. These connections allow you to share joys, concerns, and challenges with individuals who can relate to your experiences. By building these relationships, you create a community that can be a source of encouragement, advice, and lifelong connections.

In the tapestry of parenthood, building a supportive network becomes a lifeline—a source of strength, comfort, and inspiration. It is a reminder that you are never alone in this extraordinary journey. Within the intricate weave of connections, you find the encouragement to keep going, the reassurance that you are doing your best, and the affirmation that your love for your child is unwavering.

So, embrace the beauty of building a supportive network.

Chapter 6

Embracing the Changes: Physical and Emotional for Expectant Moms.

Pregnancy is a transformative journey filled with anticipation, joy, and a myriad of physical and emotional changes. As an expectant mom, understanding and embracing these changes can empower you to navigate this incredible period of your life with grace, self-compassion, and confidence. In this exploration, we will delve into the unique experiences of expectant moms, both in terms of physical transformations and emotional shifts, and discover strategies to embrace and celebrate these changes.

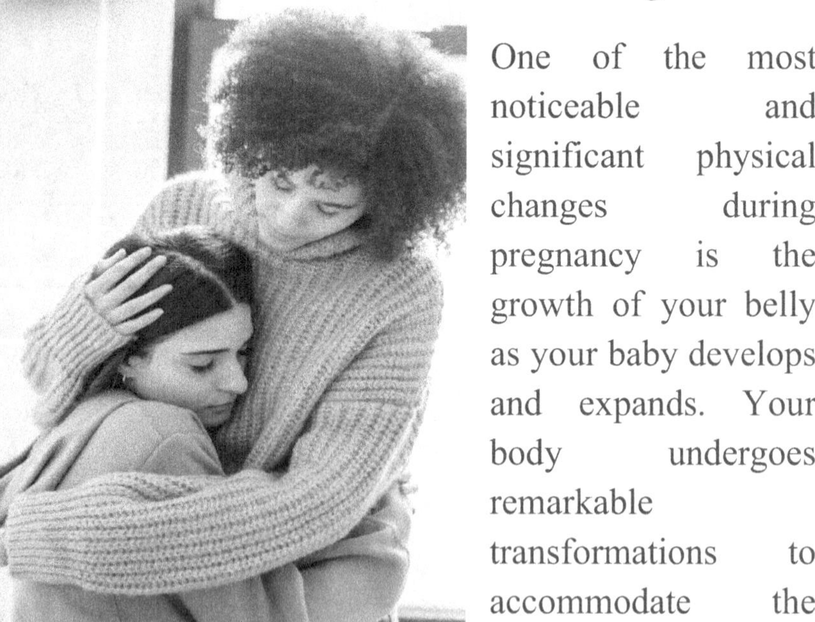

One of the most noticeable and significant physical changes during pregnancy is the growth of your belly as your baby develops and expands. Your body undergoes remarkable transformations to accommodate the growing life within you. While this is a beautiful and awe-inspiring process, it can also bring discomfort and challenges.

Embracing these physical changes begins with self-acceptance and appreciation for the incredible journey your body is undertaking. Your expanding belly is a testament to the miracle of life and the strength of your body. Celebrate and honor this transformation by embracing maternity fashion that makes you feel comfortable and beautiful. Surround yourself with supportive friends, family, and healthcare providers who can offer guidance, reassurance, and practical advice on navigating the physical changes of pregnancy. Another important physical change during pregnancy is hormonal fluctuations. Hormones play a vital role in supporting the development of your baby and preparing your body for childbirth. However, these hormonal shifts can also impact your mood, energy levels, and overall well-being. It's essential to recognize that these emotional changes are a natural part of the journey.

Embracing the emotional changes of pregnancy requires self-awareness and self-care. Listen to your body and emotions, acknowledging and honoring the range of feelings that may arise. Some days you may feel elated and connected to the new life growing inside you, while other days you may experience moments of anxiety, fear, or overwhelm. Remember that it is okay to have mixed emotions and to seek support when needed. Connect with other expectant moms, join support groups, or consider talking to a therapist who specializes in pregnancy and postpartum support. These resources can provide a safe space to share your experiences and receive guidance to navigate the emotional changes of pregnancy.

As an expectant mom, you may also experience shifts in your body image and self-esteem. The physical changes you undergo can sometimes challenge your sense of identity and impact how you perceive yourself. Embracing these changes means nurturing a positive body image and cultivating self-compassion. Focus on the incredible strength and resilience of your body. Engage in practices that promote self-care and self-love, such as gentle exercise, meditation, prenatal yoga, and nurturing skincare routines. Surround yourself with positive affirmations and reminders of the beauty and power of pregnancy. Celebrate and document the changes with maternity photoshoots or journaling, cherishing these moments as a testament to the incredible journey of motherhood.

Throughout your pregnancy, you may also encounter a wide range of expectations, opinions, and advice from others. It's important to remember that your journey is unique and deeply personal. Embracing the changes means finding the balance between seeking support and guidance from trusted sources while also listening to your intuition and making decisions that align with your values and preferences.

Educate yourself about pregnancy, childbirth, and parenting through reputable sources and seek guidance from healthcare professionals. This knowledge empowers you to make informed choices that resonate with your individual needs and desires. Surround yourself with a supportive network of friends, family, and professionals who respect your choices and provide a nurturing environment for your emotional well-being. Embracing the changes of pregnancy also involves preparing for the postpartum period and the emotions that may accompany it. The transition to motherhood brings its own set of physical and emotional changes as you adjust to the demands of caring for a newborn while recovering from childbirth. Understanding and embracing these changes can help you navigate the postpartum period with resilience and self-compassion. Physically, the postpartum period is characterized by healing and restoration. Your body goes through a process of recovery, as it gradually returns to its pre-pregnancy state. Embracing these physical changes means practicing patience and giving yourself the time and space to heal. Remember that every woman's postpartum journey is different, and there is no one-size-fits-all timeline for recovery.

Engage in gentle exercises and activities recommended by your healthcare provider to support your body's healing process. Prioritize adequate rest and nourishing meals to replenish your energy levels. Listen to your body's signals and seek support when needed, whether it's from your partner, family members, or postpartum support groups. Surround yourself with individuals who understand and validate the physical changes and challenges you may be experiencing.

Emotionally, the postpartum period can be a rollercoaster of emotions as you navigate the joys, uncertainties, and adjustments of motherhood. The hormonal fluctuations, sleep deprivation, and the demands of caring for a newborn can sometimes lead to feelings of overwhelm, exhaustion, and even postpartum mood disorders. Embracing the emotional changes of the postpartum period begins with acknowledging and accepting the wide range of emotions you may experience. It's important to remember that it's normal to feel a mix of happiness, anxiety, sadness, or frustration as you adapt to your new role as a mother. Seek support from your partner, friends, or healthcare professionals who can offer guidance and understanding during this vulnerable time.

Self-care becomes even more crucial during the postpartum period.

Carve out moments for yourself, even if they are brief, to engage in activities that bring you joy and help replenish your emotional reserves. This can include taking a relaxing bath, reading a book, going for a walk, or engaging in creative outlets such as writing or art. Remember that self-care is not selfish—it is an essential component of your well-being, allowing you to show up as the best version of yourself for your baby.

Building a support network of other mothers can also be invaluable during the postpartum period. Joining postpartum support groups or connecting with other moms through online communities can provide a sense of belonging and validation. Sharing your experiences and hearing the stories of others can help normalize the challenges and emotions you may be going through, reminding you that you are not alone on this journey.

As an expectant mom, embracing the changes—both physical and emotional—means honoring the transformative nature of pregnancy and motherhood. It means celebrating the strength and resilience of your body as it creates and nourishes life. It means cultivating self-compassion and allowing yourself the space to navigate the emotions that arise throughout this journey.

And it means seeking support, whether it's from loved ones, healthcare professionals, or fellow moms who can offer guidance and understanding.

Remember, you are embarking on an incredible and unique journey of motherhood. Embrace the changes with open arms, knowing that they are part of the profound transformation you are experiencing. Trust in your inner strength and intuition, and surround yourself with a nurturing community that can support you through the physical and emotional changes of this extraordinary time.

Embracing the changes that come with pregnancy is a journey of self-discovery, resilience, and growth. As an expectant mom, it's important to understand and navigate the physical and emotional transformations that accompany this miraculous phase of your life. By embracing these changes, you can create a nurturing environment for yourself and your growing baby. Let's explore the different aspects of embracing these changes and how they contribute to your overall well-being.

1. Physical Changes: Your body undergoes incredible transformations during pregnancy to accommodate the development of your baby. Embrace these changes as a testament to the miracle of life within you. Celebrate your growing belly, marvel at the sensations of movement, and embrace the curves and contours that showcase the strength of your body. Treat yourself to comfortable clothing that makes you feel beautiful and confident. Engage in gentle exercises, such as prenatal yoga or swimming, to stay active and maintain a healthy connection with your body.

2. Emotional Changes: Pregnancy is a time of heightened emotions and deep introspection. Your hormones may fluctuate, and you may experience a wide range of feelings, from excitement and joy to anxiety and vulnerability. Embrace these emotional changes by acknowledging and expressing your emotions without judgment. Find healthy outlets to channel your feelings, such as journaling, talking to a supportive partner or friend, or engaging in activities that bring you peace and joy. Remember that your emotional well-being is just as important as your physical health.

3. Body Image and Self-Esteem: Pregnancy can sometimes bring body image concerns and fluctuations in self-esteem. Embrace the changes by focusing on the beauty and strength of your body. Surround yourself with positive affirmations and reminders of the incredible work your body is doing. Practice self-care rituals that nurture and nourish both your body and mind, such as gentle massages, meditation, or taking quiet moments to connect with your baby. Remind yourself that you are growing a life within you, and every stretch mark and change is a badge of honor.

4. Building a Supportive Network: Surrounding yourself with a supportive network is crucial during pregnancy. Seek out other expectant moms or join prenatal support groups to connect with others who can relate to your experiences. Share your joys, concerns, and challenges with like-minded individuals who can provide guidance, empathy, and a listening ear. Your support network can be a source of comfort, inspiration, and valuable advice throughout your pregnancy journey.

5. Practicing Self-Care: Embracing the changes of pregnancy requires prioritizing self-care. Carve out time for yourself, even if it's just a few minutes each day, to engage in activities that bring you peace and rejuvenation. This can include taking warm baths, indulging in a favorite hobby, reading uplifting books, or practicing mindfulness and deep breathing exercises. Remember that taking care of yourself is not selfish but necessary for your well-being and the well-being of your baby.

6. Communication with Your Healthcare Provider: Building a trusting and open relationship with your healthcare provider is essential during pregnancy. Choose a healthcare provider who listens to your concerns, provides accurate information, and respects your choices.

Embrace open communication and ask questions about any physical or emotional changes you may be experiencing. Your healthcare provider is there to support and guide you on your journey, ensuring the best possible care for you and your baby.

7. Embracing the Unpredictable: Pregnancy is filled with surprises and the unknown. Embrace the unpredictable nature of this journey and approach it with a sense of adventure and wonder. Trust in your body's innate wisdom to nurture and protect your baby. Embrace the changes and challenges that may arise, knowing that each experience is an opportunity for growth and resilience. Have faith in your ability to adapt and navigate the unknown, and remember that you are not alone—

Physical Transformation During Pregnancy

Understanding the physical transformations during pregnancy is essential for expectant mothers. Here are some key points to help you better understand and embrace the changes that occur in your body:

1. **Weight gain:** Weight gain is a natural and necessary part of pregnancy. The recommended weight gain varies depending on your pre-pregnancy weight and individual circumstances.

It's important to focus on gaining weight gradually and maintaining a balanced, nutritious diet to support the growth and development of your baby.

2. **Hormonal changes:** Pregnancy triggers significant hormonal changes in your body. These hormonal fluctuations can cause various physical changes, such as breast enlargement and tenderness, changes in skin pigmentation, and increased vaginal discharge. Understanding that these changes are normal and temporary can help you feel more at ease.

3. **Body shape and posture:** As your baby grows, your body shape will change. Your abdomen will expand to accommodate the growing baby, and you may notice changes in your waistline and hips. These changes can affect your posture, leading to a shift in your center of gravity. It's important to practice good posture and engage in exercises that strengthen your back and core muscles to support your changing body.

4. **Breast changes:** During pregnancy, your breasts undergo changes in preparation for breastfeeding. They may become larger, more tender, and sensitive. Your nipples and areolas may darken. Wearing a well-fitting and supportive bra can help alleviate discomfort and provide necessary support.

5. **Skin changes:** Hormonal changes during pregnancy can affect your skin. Some women experience an increase in oil production, leading to acne breakouts, while others may notice changes in skin pigmentation, such as darkening of the skin in certain areas, known as melasma or the "mask of pregnancy." Additionally, stretch marks may develop as your abdomen expands. Moisturizing your skin and using sunscreen can help manage these changes.

6. **Swelling:** It's common to experience swelling, especially in the hands, feet, and ankles, during pregnancy. This is due to increased fluid retention and changes in blood circulation. Elevating your feet, wearing comfortable shoes, and avoiding prolonged periods of standing can help alleviate swelling. However, if you experience sudden or severe swelling, it's important to consult your healthcare provider.

7. **Changes in hair and nails:** Some women experience changes in hair and nail growth during pregnancy. Hair may appear thicker and shinier, while nails may grow faster. However, hormonal changes can also lead to hair loss or brittle nails for some women. Maintaining a healthy diet, practicing good hair and nail care, and being patient can help manage these changes.

8. Changes in energy levels: Pregnancy can affect your energy levels, particularly during the first and third trimesters. Fatigue and increased need for rest are common. Listen to your body and prioritize self-care by getting enough sleep, eating nutritious meals, and engaging in gentle exercise.

Remember, every pregnancy is unique, and each woman's experience may differ. It's important to consult with your healthcare provider to ensure that the physical changes you're experiencing are within the normal range. Embrace and celebrate the incredible journey of pregnancy, appreciating the remarkable transformations your body goes through to nurture and bring new life into the world.

Coping With Discomfort during Pregnancy

Coping with common discomforts during pregnancy is an important aspect of ensuring your well-being. Here are some strategies to help you find relief from common discomforts: Nausea and morning sickness:

1. **Eat small, frequent meals to prevent an empty stomach.**
   - Avoid foods and smells that trigger nausea.

- Stay hydrated by sipping on ginger tea, lemon water, or clear fluids. Get plenty of fresh air and avoid stuffy environments.
- Consider acupressure wristbands or consult your healthcare provider for safe anti-nausea remedies.

2. **Fatigue and lack of energy:**
   - Prioritize rest and aim for quality sleep.
   - Delegate tasks and ask for help from your partner, family, or friends. Incorporate gentle exercise, such as prenatal yoga or walking, to boost energy levels.
   - Eat a balanced diet rich in nutrients to support your energy levels.
   - Listen to your body and take breaks when needed.

3. **Backache and joint pain:**
   - Maintain good posture and avoid standing or sitting for extended periods.
   - Use supportive pillows while sleeping or sitting.
   - Engage in low-impact exercises, such as swimming or prenatal yoga, to strengthen core and back muscles.
   - Apply heat or cold packs to relieve discomfort.

- Consider prenatal massages or seek guidance from a physical therapist.

4. **Heartburn and indigestion:**
   - Eat smaller, more frequent meals instead of large ones.
   - Avoid spicy, fatty, and acidic foods that can trigger heartburn.
   - Sit upright for at least an hour after eating. Wear loose-fitting clothes that don't put pressure on your abdomen.
   - Consult your healthcare provider about safe antacids or other medications if needed.

5. **Swelling and fluid retention:**
   - Stay hydrated to help flush out excess fluids.
   - Avoid standing or sitting for prolonged periods.
   - Elevate your feet whenever possible.
   - Wear comfortable shoes that provide adequate support.
   - Avoid tight clothing and opt for loose-fitting, breathable fabrics.

6. **Constipation:**
   - Increase your intake of fiber-rich foods like fruits, vegetables, and whole grains.
   - Stay hydrated and drink plenty of water throughout the day.

- Engage in regular physical activity to promote healthy digestion.
- Consider stool softeners or fiber supplements after consulting with your healthcare provider.

7. **Leg cramps:**
   - Stay hydrated and drink plenty of fluids.
   - Stretch your calf muscles regularly.
   - **Avoid sitting or standing in one position for too long.**
   - Wear comfortable, supportive shoes.
   - Apply heat or massage to the affected area.

8. **Shortness of breath: Practice good posture to allow for optimal lung capacity.**
   - Avoid strenuous activities and listen to your body's signals.
   - Incorporate relaxation techniques like deep breathing and meditation.
   - Sleep in a comfortable, slightly elevated position.
   - Consult your healthcare provider if you experience severe or persistent shortness of breath.
   - Remember, every pregnancy is unique, and it's important to consult with your healthcare provider before trying any remedies or

medications, especially if you have any underlying health conditions. **They can provide personalized advice and guidance tailored to your specific needs.** Prioritizing self-care, seeking support, and communicating openly with your healthcare provider will help you cope with common discomforts and find the relief you need during this transformative time.

Emotional Changes

Addressing emotional changes during pregnancy is essential for your overall well-being. Here are some strategies to help you navigate emotional changes and seek support when needed:

1. **Acknowledge and accept your emotions:** Understand that experiencing a wide range of emotions during pregnancy is normal. Hormonal fluctuations, physical changes, and anticipation of motherhood can trigger various emotional responses. Acknowledge and accept your emotions without judgment, allowing yourself to experience and express them.

2. **Communicate with your partner:** Openly communicate with your partner about your

emotions, concerns, and needs. Sharing your feelings can strengthen your bond and help them understand what you're going through. Your partner's support and reassurance can make a significant difference in managing emotional changes.

3. **Seek support from family and friends:** Reach out to your trusted family members and friends. Share your experiences and concerns with those who can provide empathy, understanding, and a listening ear. Having a support system that validates your emotions can be comforting and reassuring.

4. **Join a prenatal support group:** Consider joining a prenatal support group where you can connect with other expectant mothers who are going through similar emotional changes. Sharing your journey, listening to others' experiences, and receiving guidance from professionals can provide a sense of camaraderie and support.

5. **Consult with a mental health professional:** If you find that your emotional changes are significantly impacting your daily life or causing distress, consider seeking help from a mental health professional, such as a therapist or counselor. They can provide guidance, tools, and

strategies to cope with emotional challenges during pregnancy.

6. **Practice self-care:** Prioritize self-care activities that promote emotional well-being. Engage in activities that you enjoy, such as reading, taking walks, practicing mindfulness or meditation, or pursuing hobbies. Take time for yourself to recharge and nurture your emotional health.

7. **Stay active and exercise:** Regular physical activity, with your healthcare provider's approval, can help alleviate stress, boost mood, and improve overall emotional well-being. Engaging in prenatal exercises, such as yoga or swimming, can provide physical and emotional benefits.

8. **Educate yourself about pregnancy and postpartum emotions:** Learn about the emotional changes that can occur during pregnancy and after childbirth. Understanding the potential challenges and knowing that others have experienced similar emotions can help normalize your feelings and provide reassurance.

9. **Be compassionate toward yourself:** Practice self-compassion and treat yourself with kindness. Pregnancy can be a time of heightened emotions and vulnerability, so it's important to be gentle with yourself. Allow yourself to rest, practice self-

care, and remind yourself that you're doing the best you can.

10. **Communicate with your healthcare provider:** Discuss your emotional changes and concerns with your healthcare provider during prenatal check-ups. They can provide guidance, resources, and potential referrals to mental health professionals if necessary. Open communication with your healthcare provider ensures that your emotional well-being is addressed as part of your overall prenatal care.

Remember, seeking support and addressing emotional changes is a sign of strength and self-care. Don't hesitate to reach out to your support network and healthcare provider when needed. Your emotional well-being is just as important as your physical health during pregnancy, and by addressing your emotions and seeking support, you can navigate this transformative time with greater resilience and positivity.

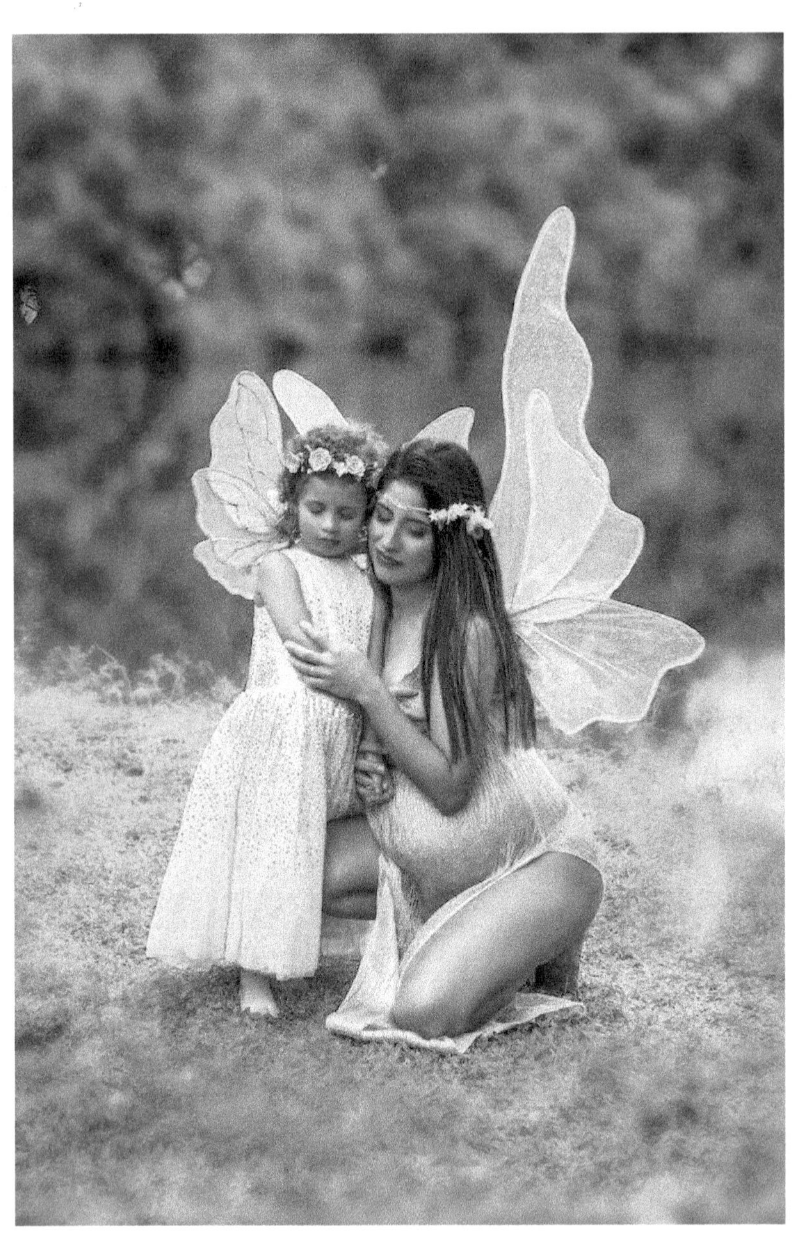